Tamilee Webb's
Defy Gravity Workout

Tamilee Webb's
Defy Gravity Workout

The Revolutionary Program
That Lifts and Tones Your Entire Body

Tamilee Webb
with Cheryl Fenton

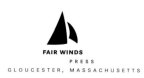

FAIR WINDS
PRESS
GLOUCESTER, MASSACHUSETTS

First published in the USA in 2005 by
Fair Winds Press
33 Commercial Street
Gloucester, MA 01930

08 07 06 05 04   1 2 3 4 5

ISBN 1-59233-087-8

Library of Congress Cataloging-in-Publication Data available

Cover and book design by
Laura H. Couallier, Laura Herrmann Design

Printed and bound in Singapore

*The information in this book is for educational purposes only.
It is not intended to replace the advice of a physician or medical practitioner.
Please see your health care provider before beginning any new health program.*

DEDICATION

This book is dedicated to my family—Mom, Barbara J. Webb,
and my two brothers, Ronny W. Webb and Rodney G. Webb
(in spite of making fun of my bubble butt)
for their constant love and support!

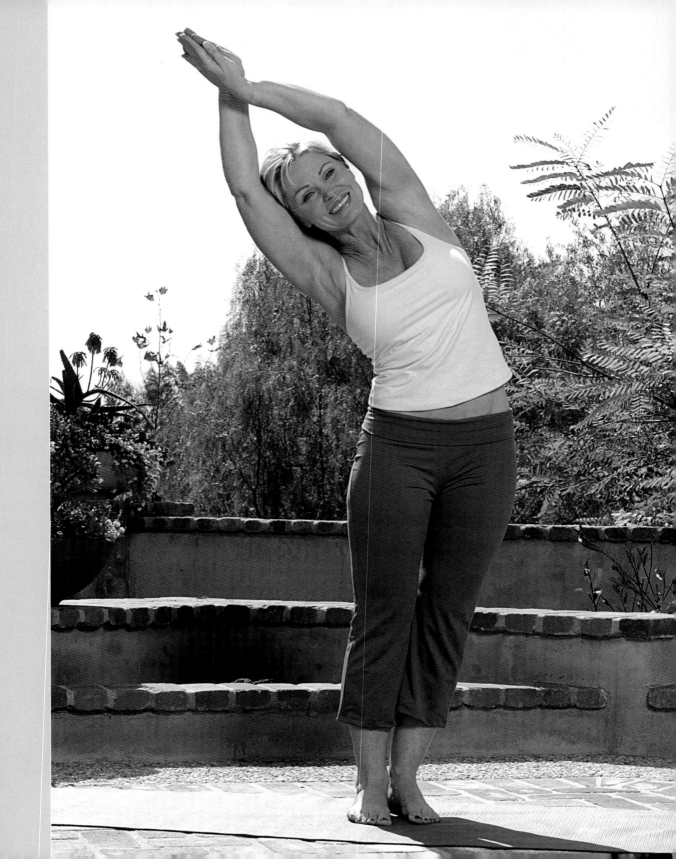

Contents

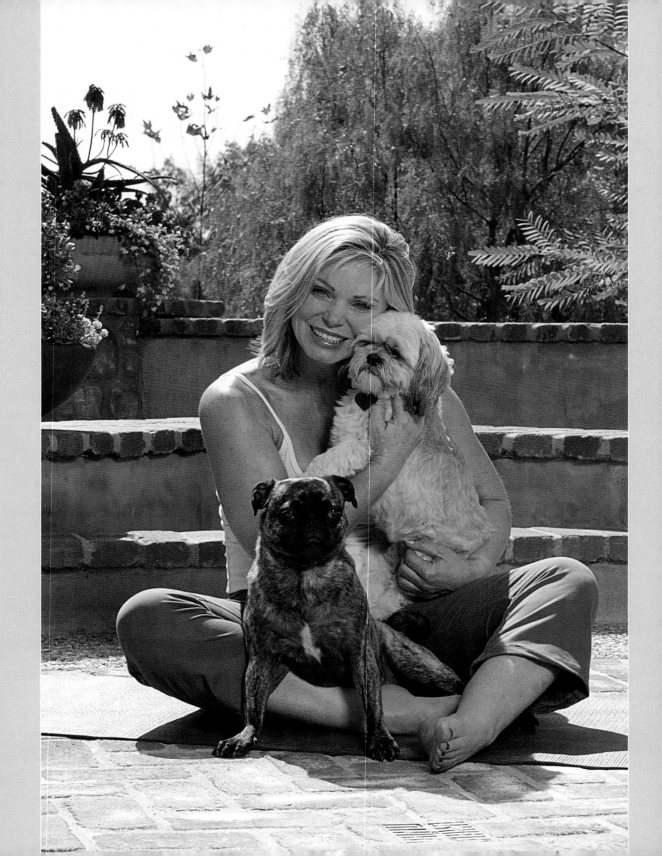

Introduction

What Happened to My Buns and Abs of Steel?

Have you ever seen pictures of yourself from ten years ago and thought, "My body wasn't so bad back then." The ironic part is that at that time, you were convinced that you could probably stand to lose a few pounds. A decade later, you are now realizing that you would kill to have that body back.

That's how I feel when I look back at the *Buns of Steel* videos I made in my thirties. When I look at them now, I ask myself, "What was I thinking?" I was so hard on myself back then and I looked so good! Of course, it's easy to be tough on yourself when you're in the fitness industry, like I am. But, as a fitness leader, it was important that I represent a physical and professional ideal to the best of my ability and what I was representing at the time was…a body of steel!

Now, in my forties, I'm learning ways to love and accept my body, even though it is more difficult today to keep myself fit, strong, and in tip-top condition than it was ten years ago.

But why is it so much harder? What makes the body of a twenty-year-old so much easier to maintain than the mature shape of a forty-year-old? Well, the culprits are age and gravity. We don't think we have the weight of the world on us until we see that it has been pulling and tugging on our face and body. What was once sitting high up north is now sagging down south.

And society certainly doesn't know how to forgive and forget when it comes to your aging body. Living in a world that doesn't accept women aging gracefully is like driving in a neighborhood full of dead end streets—you don't know which way to turn. From our skin to our hair to the inevitable weight gain, women feel the brunt of this scrutiny as their age creeps up in years. Men can have salt-and-pepper hair and still be considered sexy; but how many women do you see on the evening news or in advertisements with even a touch of gray?

We are constantly told by the media and Hollywood what to wear, how to look, what to do if you don't have it, and then where to find what they think you need. Don't get me wrong, I'm guilty of looking through the pages of fashion magazines to see who is wearing what and when. I love fashion and want to look my best, but let's get real…life is more than working out with your trainer, putting on the most expensive outfit, and getting your nails and hair done on the way to cocktails with the girls.

In our twenties we are youthful, full of energy, and thinking only of our next date. We are untouchable, lying in the sun frying our faces and bodies, and partying all night. We don't think twice about going to bed without washing our makeup off. And yet we still manage to jump up out of bed the next day looking great while running off to class or work. The gym is someplace that we visit only when we have the time (but who has the time?). Besides, we have so many other things to "conquer," and our physiques don't seem to notice that lack of exercise.

You start out happy that you have no hips or boobs.
All of a sudden you get them, and it feels sloppy.
Then just when you start liking them, they start dropping.

—Cindy Crawford

Our thirties bring us to a new level of awareness. We find ourselves waking out of the daydream with the "Oh my gosh, I can't believe I'm turning thirty" worry and "the clock is ticking" mantra. And either we're on a mission to find the man of our dreams or to climb the ladder of success in our career, or both. Our paces pick up while our metabolism slows down, leaving us with less energy to party all night or hit the gym for a quick workout. Long hours at work or chasing after the kids is about all the energy we can muster. It's only when we try to fit into our favorite jeans (the ones that once slid right over our hips) that we realize that our body is changing. This is where we get caught up in the five- to ten-pound roller coaster ride. By our late thirties, a couple of kids, a few yo-yo diets, and hundreds of workouts later, we begin to panic because the big 4-0 is around the corner.

We grow neither better nor worse as we get old, but more like ourselves.

—Mary Lambertson Becker

Like most women, I dreaded turning forty. After all, it is such a big turning point in one's life. After the panic passes and you start to settle into your own, you become aware that there are even more hurdles to clear: your metabolism dropping, weight increasing, bone density decreasing, hormones flying every which way, getting out of bed in the morning taking a little longer, and Advil becoming a daily self-medication. And you can always spot a woman in her early forties… she holds menus and newspapers at a distance—a dead give-away! This is the beginning of changes called perimenopause, the time when your body is getting ready to go into menopause. Since I'm an expert about going through it, but not about explaining it, I recommend reading up on the matter (see the Resources section).

Welcome to the Age of Defying Gravity

I've written this book to try and help women like us fight the battle against gravity. From tips on choosing the right beauty regimen to the healthiest snacks, along with easy-to-follow exercise routines, I hope I help you look years younger and feel great.

Many women would much rather be thinner than live longer, according to a survey in *Psychology Today.* This doesn't have to be the case. There are ways to both live longer and be happy with our bodies. If you're a woman approaching your forties or fifties, then you're reading anything and everything you can get your hands on to defy gravity and fight the battle against aging. From my extensive research to interviewing friends and clients about their personal experiences, as well as information from my own life discoveries, I am here to share all I have found with you.

I look forward to being older, when what you look like becomes less and less an issue and what you are is the point.

—Susan Sarandon

As a woman who appears on videos and television at times, I feel the pressure of society to look as perfect as possible no matter what it takes. If I'm feeling this way, how do you think the real stars in Hollywood are feeling? Most will go to extremes to keep themselves looking young and their body parts staying where they were in their twenties. Have you ever noticed they all have the same nose, boobs, and look on their face?

I think a woman's looks shouldn't be cookie-cutter, but individual! Too many times I hear women talking about their bodies, focusing on what they don't like rather than what they do like. I know women who won't gain an ounce because they think their husbands would leave them if they gained weight. So they starve themselves, exercise like crazy, and wear ridiculous clothes that only Britney Spears should be wearing…certainly not a forty-something woman!

Somewhere along the way, our society got caught up on how we look on the outside. My opinion on this matter is that it's because we are very visual beings. No one would ever praise you (unless it's your doctor) for a lovely liver, a healthy heart, or clear lungs. If people could "unzip" themselves, don't you think they'd take better care of their bodies? Most of us take better care of our cars than we do of our bodies, probably because we can open up their hoods and take a look inside at the engine.

My philosophy toward fitness is simple. Fitness begins from within—your brain, heart, lungs, blood, muscles, and all your internal organs—then works its way to the outside. Your healthy looks and toned body are your reward for taking care of your health. If you take care of yourself for your health, not necessarily your looks, then you'll be fit. This is because everything on the inside of our bodies needs proper exercise, nutrition, and rest in order to function at full force.

To dream too much of the person you would like to be is to waste the person you are.

—Anonymous

Measuring Body Fat–
It's Size, Not Weight, That Matters

When I see an overweight person, I don't look at them as a fat person. I see an unhealthy body that needs education, love, and support toward a healthier lifestyle. It is hard living in a world where slim is "in."

There is overweight, then there is obesity. If a person is overweight, it means their body fat is above the recommended range for good health, whereas obesity means someone is severely overweight with an accumulation of body fat of more than 33% (in women). This creates a higher health risk than just being overweight.

**FEMALE PERCENT
BODY FAT CLASSIFICATION**

Percent Body Fat	Classification
Less then 8%	Excessively lean
8–19%	Lean
20–30%	Acceptable
31–33%	Borderline obese
More than 33%	Obese

(*Fit & Well*, page 139, table 6-1)

There are many ways to measure your body fat—Body Mass Index, Caliper Skin Fold, Hydrostatic (underwater) Weighing, and Bioelectrical Impedance Analysis (BIA). Knowing your ratio of lean body mass to body fat is more important than your total body weight, which is what most of us mistakenly focus on. But scales can only tell you your total body weight at that moment, and sometimes what you see as extra pounds is really water weight. It's the fat on our body that we should be concerned about! This goes back to what we can't see from the inside of our body. Don't think because someone is slim they are fit and healthy. You can be thin and still not be healthy. There are many different body types but all types have one thing in common…they require exercise!

Body Mass Index (BMI)

Your BMI is calculated by:

$$\text{BMI} = \frac{\text{weight in lbs} \times 703}{(\text{height in inches}) \times (\text{height in inches})}$$

Calipers Skin Fold

Calipers are instruments with two jaws that can be adjusted to determine thickness of skin folds in various sites on your body.

Hydrostatic Weighing

With this method, you sit on a harness device that is connected to a scale in a large tank of water. You are asked to take a deep breath in and exhale out as much air as you can as you are lowered underwater. The percentages of fat and fat-free weight are calculated from body density…fat floats, muscle sinks.

Bioelectrical Impedance Analysis (BIA)

This type of test works by sending a small electrical current through your body and measuring your body's resistance to it. There are scales sold that measure BIA.

It's Never About the Scale

When thinking about the state of their bodies, most women focus on the number on the scale, but, really, it's clothing size (or tape measure numbers) that is a better indicator of your health. Not every woman has to be a size four, of course, but if your clothing size has crept up over the years then there is a good chance you want to defy gravity.

Maybe you're wondering just why we expand as the years go by. Well, when we're young, our bodies have lots of muscle, even if we don't work out, and muscle takes up less space than fat. The ironic thing is that muscles weigh more than fat, so, in the long run, changes in numbers on the scale might not tell you much about your health. It might be better for you to judge how you feel in your clothes than look at the scale to determine if you want to change the way you look.

That's why the promise of this book is to drop two dress sizes in eight weeks—because if you lose fat through cardio exercise and eating well, but gain muscle with strength-training, you may not actually lose that much weight (in pounds) but you will change the shape of your body and be able to wear smaller-sized clothes.

Quick Tips on Defying Gravity

* **Take Care of Your Body:** That means as a whole—mentally, physically, and spiritually!

* **Exercise:** Be active! The exercises in the *Defy Gravity Workout* have been selected to best defy gravity by strengthening, toning, and shaping your muscles.

* **Eat Healthy:** Eating foods that are rich in antioxidants are better for your skin, cells, and body. Think organic, non-chemical foods that are not loaded with toxins. Eat fewer calories.

* **Protect Yourself from the Sun:** Sun is the quickest way to lose firmness in your skin. Always wear sunscreen or some form of protection against direct sunlight. Treat your skin to a daily cleansing, moisturizer, and sunscreen. Your skin needs a health program just like your body.

* **Get Plenty of Rest:** Your body needs rest to repair itself. Also, a rested mind is a happy mind that can think more clearly and has more energy.

* **Keep Your Mind Sharp and Positive:** Active minds are more likely to remain healthy.

* **Don't Smoke!** Smoking is not only bad for your lungs, it is also damaging to your skin, eventually giving it a dry, wrinkled, and saggy look.

These lifestyle and health changes begin now, so let's get started.

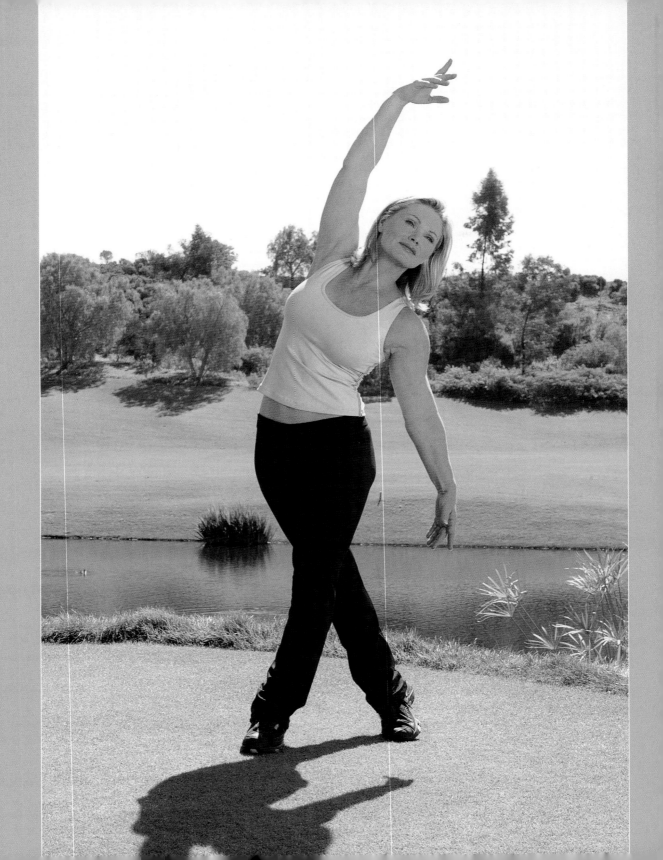

CHAPTER ONE

Getting Started

From our bodies to our looks to our attitude,
*we are **what** and **how much** we eat.*

Nutrition

Eating for Your Age and Health

Nutrition is a vital component to protecting ourselves against disease and other health problems. How much and what we should eat varies as we age. But no matter how old we are, our bodies require a balance of vitamins and nutrients, protein, carbohydrates, and fats.

Unfortunately, sometimes the food we eat doesn't actually feed us with nutrients; instead, it gives us calories in the forms of fat and sugar, but no vitamins or minerals. Living in a society that is all about fast paced, fast food and a world that is all about convenience makes it hard to slow down and take time to fuel up on whole foods. Have you ever felt sluggish or low on energy? It could be because you need to refuel your body with some nutrients. Food gives us the fuel to keep going. When we feel that first drag of low energy, some of us reach for a quick fix, like caffeine or sugar for a speedy boost of energy. The problem is that this briefly takes our energy up and then it drops us back down because the choice of nutrients wasn't the right choice.

Your Mid-Life Nutritional Needs

Based on what your daily routine and age are, you'll need to make nutritional changes throughout your life. This is especially important for women thirty-five years of age and older who are experiencing hormonal changes. As women, our hormone estrogen decreases later in life, creating changes to our metabolism, fat cells, emotions, and body temperature. This is a wake-up call, because even though you're doing everything the same—exercising, eating healthy, and getting plenty of rest—no matter what you do, your results will change. You won't lose weight so easily. What was once an old friend that you knew so well is now a body you don't know at all. Learning to understand what is happening to your middle-aged body is the first step to getting it all back under control. It used to be that your forties were considered middle-aged. I don't believe this is true in today's world. The forties are the new thirties, the fifties the new forties, and so on. Thanks to better living, healthy attitudes, and medical technology, we are living longer today than we did forty years ago. However, that doesn't mean a woman's hormonal changes will be delayed. But these days, we are better educated when it comes to menopause or perimenopause and how to handle these changes wisely.

How you go through these changes and the outcome depends a great deal on your attitude, fitness, nutrition, and lifestyle. No one knows this better than Debra Waterhouse, author, nutrition expert, registered dietitian, and mother. I learned about Debra from her book *Outsmarting the Female Fat Cell,* which I love and recommend to my clients. Her *Outsmarting the Mid-Life Fat Cell* deals with how women's metabolisms change as they age. I don't claim to be an expert on nutrition, but I do know all the basics—what is clean, healthy eating and what isn't. Debra tells it like it really is—no fluff, no lies. I like that approach and I consider it similar to my workout programs. For more information, see the resources section.

Nutrition and a woman's fat cells go hand-in-hand (or should I say mouth-to-fat cell). My fat cells at age forty-five are different than they were in my twenties or early thirties…these days, they are stubborn! Fat cells produce estrogen with age and help us with menopause. What I could eat when I was young has changed because my fat cells now prefer to store rather than release fat. And their favorite place to store is around my waistline and arms. How much I eat has also changed. We have "supersized" everything in America, and that needs to change. Our portions should not be any bigger than the palm of one hand, which is about the size of one's stomach.

Understanding fat cells and how they can benefit us in a positive way through nutrition and exercise is an important step in the success of reaching realistic goals at any age. Because my metabolism is ten to fifteen percent slower than it was a few years ago, I need to eat less and exercise more. I know some of you reading this might be getting discouraged with what seems to be bad news about aging, but don't be. If you're prepared and educated on the matter, it should be a piece of cake (just a smaller piece)!

Free Radicals

Who said nothing is free? Free radicals are! These are molecules of oxygen that have lost an electron in a chemical reaction that damages cell membranes. Think of them as cling-ons…aliens looking for a place to invade. Once they "cling-on" to an electron (which can be anything from our DNA to fats and proteins produced through exposure to environmental factors like sunlight or smog), they damage our cells. Antioxidants and nutrients are the fighting substances that can prevent free radicals from damaging our DNA. Here are a few tips on protecting against free radicals:

* Eat a balanced diet that contains foods rich in antioxidants, vitamins, and minerals.
* Avoid smoking and second-hand smoke.
* Reduce your intake of fat and salt.
* Exercise regularly.

In order to build our immune system, it's important to include foods rich in nutrients. The foods we choose can also significantly affect our risk of cancer. Eating five to nine servings of fruits and vegetables per day ensures a diet high in fiber and rich in cancer-fighting phytochemicals (*phyto* means plant).

We are exposed to over 10,000 new chemicals each year through processed foods. Processed foods contain preservatives and chemicals and affect our body internally by being harder to digest and causing gastrointestinal stress. Eating natural or organic foods (without any chemicals or preservatives) is best for our body. Sometimes we don't eat the recommended foods needed in our diet. This is where taking vitamins and minerals can help optimize our health.

The following is a recommended "over-forty" dietary supplement guide from *Fight Fat After Forty* by Pamela Peeke, M.D..

RECOMMENDED OVER-FORTY DIETARY SUPPLEMENTS

- **Multivitamin and mineral***
  supplement
- **Vitamin E:** 400 IU (up to 800 IU if heart disease is present or risk is high)
- **Selenium:** 100 mcg (up to 200 mcg is immune system is compromised)
- **Vitamin C:** 250 mg (up to 500 mg if at high risk for heart disease or 1,000 mg if heart disease is present)
- **Vitamin B complex**
- **Calcium:** 1,000–1,500
- **Vitamin D:** 200 IU (only if not included in multivitamin or calcium supplement)
- **Omega (fish) Oil:** 1,000 mg
- **Flaxseed Oil:** 1,000 mg

* *Multivitamins should contain 100% of established value of vitamins and minerals*

Adopt a Healthy Eating Habit
Each Week with Defy Gravity

If you struggle with your weight because of poor eating habits, I've created an easy way for you to improve. In each week of Defy Gravity, I'll suggest a new habit for you to try out. Of course, I hope you'll keep each habit during the following weeks, so that by the end of the program you will have a whole new way of eating.

I want to reassure you that this doesn't mean you will have to give up your favorite treats. If it's important to you that you have chocolate every few days (or even every day) then you will be able to do that. I would suggest that you focus on proper portions (a piece of chocolate isn't going to make anyone fat, but a few candy bars a day will) and also on making healthy choices (you'll see that it's better to eat chocolate that isn't made with hydrogenated oils or high fructose corn syrup).

Meanwhile, if you've adopted other healthy eating habits, such as eating enough fruits and vegetables and choosing lean proteins, then the proper portion of chocolate won't be such a big deal in the long run.

SOME OF MY FAVORITE MEALS AND SNACKS

- **Breakfast**

  Oatmeal, scrambled egg whites with veggies, 1/2 banana or a couple of strawberries, 1 cup of coffee, and water

  Yogurt (low fat) with bran cereal mixed in it

  1 slice of whole wheat bread with 1/2 tsp. of peanut butter spread on it and 1/2 cup of hot natural applesauce poured over it...yum

- **Lunch**

  Salad with chicken and low-fat vinaigrette dressing

  Wild salmon, grilled vegetables and brown rice

  Tuna mixed with low fat cottage cheese

  Veggie wrap made with a whole wheat tortilla, lean turkey, low-fat cheese, lettuce, tomato, and vinaigrette dressing

- **Dinner**

  Wild salmon over butter lettuce with a little blue cheese sprinkled on top

  Grilled chicken breast and veggie salad with vinaigrette dressing

  Baked or grilled vegetables with a little olive oil

  Tofu, broccoli, sobe noodles, and fat-free chicken broth

- **Snack Options**

  Ten almonds, low-fat Ritz crackers, low-fat cottage cheese and fruit, corn tortilla with chicken breast and salsa, half a protein bar with fruit, sliced turkey, baby carrots, hard boiled eggs (just whites), air popped popcorn, salt-free pretzels, celery with organic low-fat peanut butter, low-fat cheese, nonfat yogurt

Learn to Cope Well with Stress

Stress is a common word in today's conversation. Most of us are stressed out about something, and we all have our own ways of coping. Research has discovered that women are more sensitive to stress than men. Women and men also cope with stress differently. Men are more likely to turn to alcohol, while women will seek social support from others. Women on an average live seven and a half years longer than men, so maybe these hormones that cause so much trouble at times really do help us live longer.

Scientists have come up with the well-known phrases "fight or flight" and "tend and befriend" to describe responses to stress. Most of the early research on stress was done on males, where it was discovered that men are more likely to fight or flight in a stressful situation. Later on, females were included in research. It was found that most females will protect their young, make friends, create bonds, or develop a social network—or "tend and befriend."

Stressful situations trigger physical and emotional reactions, leading to symptoms that show up either immediately or later. Emotionally, stress causes bad moods, a short temper, and maybe even a little snacking when we aren't really hungry. But, even more importantly, stress takes a physical toll on your body.

The nervous and endocrine systems are the two major systems that respond physically to stress. The nervous system relates to the brain, spinal cord, and nerves, while the endocrine system relates to the glands, tissues, and cells that help control body functions by releasing hormones and other chemical messengers into the blood stream. By depending on these two systems, your body prepares itself for stress. The hormones released during stress are cortisol, epinephrine, and norepinephrine. These trigger physiological changes in hearing, vision, heart rate, perspiration, and energy.

You've heard of the endorphins that runners get sometimes that produce a "runners high." This is a time when you feel like you can do anything because your reflexes and strength are heightened. This is a great example showing us there are both good and bad stressors. It works the same way if you find yourself in a dangerous situation. Going into depth about this subject would take up volumes, but you can read more about these stress factors in *Fit & Well,* a book by one of my favorite professors, Dr. Thomas D. Fahey, Ph.D.

When we exercise, we stress our body, but it's a beneficial stress that is good for us. On the other hand, we can have negative stress when we go through a tragedy, like losing a loved one or going through a divorce. I learned it first hand when my father died of a heart attack when I was fourteen and with my divorce two years ago. These were events that affected me both emotionally and physically.

In response to these stressful situations, my body went into survival mode. I couldn't eat, sleep, concentrate, or control my emotions. Eventually, I gained weight. I even ended up on anti-depression medication and other drugs to help me sleep. Those who know me were surprised to see this strong, independent, outgoing woman change. To be honest, so was I. During this time I mostly didn't like being me nor did I want others to be around me. Deep down I knew I had the power to change my attitude, but I also knew I had to go through certain emotions to heal.

My friend Tami once gave me a beautiful framed poem for my birthday. It read:

A POSITIVE ATTITUDE

Our lives are not determined by what happens to us, but by how we react to what happens; not by what life brings us, but by the attitude we bring to life. A positive attitude causes a chain reaction of positive thoughts, events and outcomes. It is a catalyst… A spark that creates extraordinary results.

—Unknown

To this day I keep it on my dresser and read it every day as a reminder that it is up to me how I respond to whatever comes my way, be it a distressing event or a stressful situation. I cannot change what happens, but I can change how I respond to it. Thank you, Tami, for that lesson!

When a person is under pressure, their body releases the stress hormone cortisol, which stimulates the uptake of fat into abdominal fat cells. Under stress as a woman now in her mid-forties, this is when I realized my "Abs of Steel" had jumped ship and were nowhere to be found. It's common for men and women to develop a "spare tire" around the middle during midlife. So now I've gone through a divorce, moved, and begun midlife. After realizing that I can control my stress level, I say, "Bring it on!" because I know that I can de-stress myself through exercise, healthy eating, meditation, and the love and support from family and friends. (That's another entire unexpected wake up call. You really learn who your true friends are when you go through a life change. If it's said that friends are a reflection of a person, then I'm doing great. I have the best girlfriends in the world and because of their love and support I was able to de-stress my situation. Thanks, girls. I love you!)

If I wasn't known as the "Buns of Steel" woman, I wouldn't think twice about the little roll I have around my waist. I'd be looking pretty good for a woman of my age! But I am that woman and I live in Southern California where fitness and bikinis are everywhere. I don't believe there ever comes a time when a woman says she completely and totally loves her body just as it is, but I think we can come to accept the things we cannot change with age.

The body manifests what the mind harbors.
—Jerry Augustine

We all deal with stress in different ways—some through food, others with alcohol, drugs, self abuse or isolation, and depression. Each one of these responses is unhealthy to the body. There truly is a connection between mind and body. Thinking positively has been touted as a great way to battle stress because it works. What you think can manifest into physical form. If you're always thinking bad thoughts and acting very "woe is me," then that is going to manifest itself in your health. Healthy positive minds mean a healthier body. My (ex) father-in-law, whom I continue to call "Dad," has the most positive outlook on life at 80 years old. Whenever I ask him, "How are you doing, Dad?" his answer has always been, "Fannnntastic!" Whether he is really feeling great or not, you believe him because of his smile and the tone of his voice. People love to be around others who are happy and full of life and energy! This positive energy and attitude spread to others, and we all want it! So when someone asks me how I'm doing, I always think of the man who taught me to respond with an attitude that everyone loves to hear…Fannntasic! (Thank you, Dad Chasan.)

So it's up to you how you cope with stress. But know this—you better get it under control before it takes over and controls you. Learn to handle stress before it gets a (love) handle on you! Here are some guaranteed stress busters:

* **Exercise**—Think of it as an insurance policy that will keep you fit and healthy for a longer life.

* **Positive Attitude**—Stop the negative thoughts and replace them with positive ones. Be optimistic with a positive outlook.

* **Eat Healthy**—When the body receives the nutrients it needs, it can better cope with stress.

* **Support**—Talk to your friends or professionals who can help you work through difficult times.

* **Meditation**—By quieting the mind, the body relaxes, breathing slows down, and blood flows to the brain—all of this helps us to calm, clear our minds, and release stress.

* **Time Management**—By having a schedule, you can set priorities and accomplish your tasks within the time allotted. Don't over-schedule yourself and stick to your plan.

* **Rest**—Getting seven to eight hours of rest repairs your body, rejuvenating it and allowing for better mental and physical responses.

Remember, your health is dependent on your ability to eat healthy, exercise regularly, and cope with any kind of stress that comes your way! Take a deep breath, clear your mind, and learn to let it all go.

The Importance of Variety

Variety is the spice of life. It keeps us from boredom no matter what we're doing. The same goes for our muscles. They need variety to stay "interested" and work at their full potential. Once a muscle repeats a movement over and over, it becomes familiar with the action and goes through the motion without any thought. When it's required to perform a movement or contraction that is different than usual, it will respond by calling in all the motor nerves and muscle fibers, saying, "Hey guys, this is new! Wake up!" This explains why you feel sore the next day after a new workout. Your muscles had to work harder than usual and now need twenty-four hours to recover before the next workout.

There is a good reason I have selected walking, muscle training, yoga, and Pilates as the Defy Gravity Workout. They give you a balanced variety workout that will help you defy gravity. These exercises are gentler to your joints, but still give you the benefits you crave. Why do you think yoga and Pilates have made such a come back? They've been around for ages, but today's fitness crowd is full of baby boomers who are continuing to exercise in their mid-life. Yoga and Pilates give you more than just jumping up and down in an aerobics class or running on the hard pavement. They allow you to go deeper than the surface—breathing deeply and slowly, feeling the body stretch or bend into positions you never thought possible.

Walking works because it is an activity everyone can do. What I love most about it is the intervals. My mesomorph body isn't built for long-distance running and I find my hips begin to hurt after a mile of jogging. With Interval Walking Workouts, you can walk or jog for three minutes knowing that at the end of those three minutes you get a two-minute recovery. This keeps you motivated and your body from fatiguing too quickly, as it would if you were just jogging. The other advantage is your heart works harder because of the fast and slow paces. You're burning fat and calories, as well as getting muscle benefits—especially in your legs, calves, and butt.

After the age of thirty, we lose muscle mass. This slows down our metabolism, which in turn will increase our body fat if we're inactive. Although men generally have larger muscles than women, both sexes need to keep muscles strong to offset osteoporosis, keep motor nerves connected, and help prevent injuries as we age.

The exercises in the Muscle Training Workout are designed to strengthen and tighten your muscles and keep them guessing. Every two weeks the exercises change to challenge your muscles and increase the intensity of the workout. Some of the exercises will combine core work with a specific muscle, such as the one-legged, one-arm bicep curl. Standing on one leg while doing a bicep curl will engage your core (abdominal and lower back) muscles to help balance and stabilize your body while curling your arm up and down.

There are many other activities to choose from, and I encourage you to mix it up and keep your fitness program fresh and your muscles guessing. The bottom line is to keep moving. Once you stop, you lose what you gained more quickly than you worked to get it. It's harder to get back into a routine than staying with it. If you're someone who starts a new program every New Year's Day, think back to how you feel the first couple of weeks of exercising—you're sore, maybe you have blisters. That kinda makes it hard to get up and do it again, doesn't it? But this passes with each time you get up and do it, so if you stay in a routine, you will start seeing benefits. And just as the seasons change, so should your workouts. Take care of your body and your body will take care of you!

What You Need To Defy Gravity

Time is the most important ingredient to make this program work for you. Plan on spending sixty minutes, six days a week. Some of you might be thinking there is no way you can squeeze sixty minutes into your day to do something just for yourself. After all, that would be selfish—the kids need to be taken here and there, the laundry needs to be done, and what about preparing dinner? I answer you with another question: If you were so sick that you couldn't get out of bed, who would take care of all your daily chores? You would need to arrange help to deal with all the home management and kids, right? That's my point. Why not take care of yourself, so you're not in that situation too often? Taking care of yourself should be your number one priority. If you're healthy, you can do all the things that your family is counting on you to do.

After you make the time, the next thing you'll need to begin your program is a good pair of **walking shoes** (see Walking Basics in chapter 2 for tips on choosing the right shoe), along with comfortable clothing that allows free movement and is made of fabric that breathes. Other than that, equipment is minimal and optional for most of the routines. I suggest **dumbbells, a mat, a step or bench, and a stop watch or second-hand watch** for the walking intervals. All of these are available online or at your local sporting goods store and shouldn't cost you a fortune. So shop around and find the best deal.

The hand weights or dumbbells should be between two to ten pounds, heavier if you're an experienced exerciser. Don't be afraid of heavy weights; they won't give you big bulky muscles. Women aren't genetically predisposed to having the large muscles of a man. The dumbbells I'm using in the photos throughout the book are from Nike and are a good choice for a cushioned, hand-held weight. The step I'm using is from the Step Company.

There are many affordable sport watches in the market that will not only give you the time, but also calories burned, heart rate, and distance. Mio is my favorite watch because it doesn't require you to have a strap around your chest to take your heart rate.

The last thing you'll need for a successful workout is an attitude that you deserve to have a fit, lean healthy body to take you to eternity and beyond.

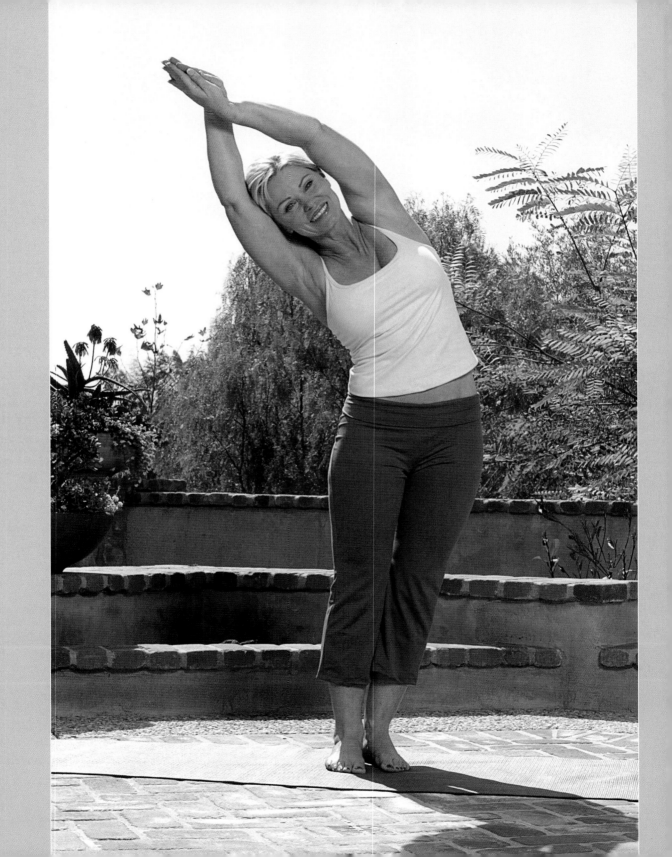

CHAPTER TWO

The Basics

Walking Basics

Walking is as easy as putting on a pair of sneakers and walking out the door of your house or office building. And it is one of the most beneficial workouts because it also helps with improving your mood, warding off depression, lowering high blood pressure, decreasing your chances of heart disease, helping with weight loss, giving anti-aging benefits, promoting bone formation and tissue regeneration—the list goes on and on.

But form certainly precedes function in this case. From what to wear to the right fuel for a great workout, there are a few things you should know before you get started.

The Gear You'll Need

Shoes are the most important consideration when it comes to walking. And as the options are limitless when it comes to choices, there are certain guidelines to follow for the perfect fit. Investment is important, so if you can, choose a well-made shoe that might come with a higher price tag. Cheap shoes may cost you less money, but they will cost you plenty in the health of your feet and back. Good walking shoes can run from about fifty dollars on up. Don't be afraid to ask the salesperson questions about the quality of the shoe, support, cushioning, and personal recommendations.

The biomechanics of walking are different than other sports, even running. So you need footwear that is designed with those differences in mind. Walking is a linear movement, so your heels pay the price. Your shoes also must allow your feet flexibility, so that they roll properly. This is different from other activities, like aerobics, which is lateral and needs more cushioning on the forefoot than the heel, or running, which needs less flexibility and heel cushioning.

Here's what to look for when buying a walking shoe:

1. Make sure that the shoe feels resilient when you land on your heel. It shouldn't wobble and it should fit snugly around your heel.

2. A roomy toe box will give you plenty of space to allow your toes to spread as you push off the ground with each step. A rule of thumb—you need half a thumb's distance from your big toe to the tip of the shoe.

3. Look for forefoot flexibility by bending the shoe. A stiff shoe might cause shin pain.

4. Choose low heels over chunky heels. This will give you less weight to crash your foot down with, which forces your shin muscles to work harder to brake the action.

5. Choose lightweight for speed and ease in your workout.

6. Look for mesh that will allow your feet to air out and release heat.

Try both shoes on and take time to walk around the store in them to get a feel for how they fit your feet. And a word to the wise, don't use new shoes if you are planning on going for a long walk. Brand new walking shoes typically need a period of breaking in, so try wearing them for a quick trip around the mall or to run errands before using them for workouts.

If your socks aren't the proper type, you won't get the most benefit from your shoes. And don't be fooled by cheap socks. You'll only get a few good wears out of them before they start falling apart from washing and usage. Also be wary of thin socks, which can give you blisters and begin to rub in certain areas. Buy socks that are thick cotton or wool, as they will wick away sweat and keep your feet dry and cushioned.

Other clothing depends on the weather. If it's cold and damp outside, be sure to layer. Begin with a thin layer, such as exercise tights made of fabric that dries quickly (avoid cotton). The next layer should be pieces that will insulate your body, such as a fleece sweatshirt. To keep the damp at bay, finish up with a water-resistant jacket. The rest is common sense. If your hands get cold, try thin gloves. For cold ears, try earmuffs or a headband. And if you are lucky enough to be taking advantage of a beautiful day, walking shorts (something with a range of movement), a T-shirt (a dry weave is best for sweat), and a support sports bra are the ticket. And don't ever forget the last layer—whether cloudy or clear, wear sunscreen (more on this in chapter 4)!

We've covered what goes onto your body. But what about what goes in it? First and foremost, never forget water. Even without working out, our bodies need at least sixty-four ounces of water daily. When you are exercising and working up a sweat, you will need even more to replenish your body's supply. A rule to remember…if you're thirsty, you are already dehydrated. So start drinking. Take along a water bottle or two on your walk. For an added workout, use them as if they were dumbbells; just make sure you drink them equally during the workout to keep the weight balanced.

Now that you know what to wear and what to bring, where do you go? Should you hit the road or watch your favorite show while you pound the "pavement" on a treadmill? This is up to you, whatever you prefer, though you can decide based on the weather or season. There are pros and cons to both. The obvious price issue aside, treadmills are convenient, offer great variations for inclines and speed, and you can walk on them during even the rainiest or snowiest of weather. But, on the other hand, they take up space (if in your home), have limited views (unless set up right in front of a television), and you have to walk or jog when it's on. Walking without a treadmill requires self-motivation; it's up to you to move, to change speed, duration, and intensity of workout. It's less expensive than a treadmill (unless you count the cost for good shoes), offers fresh air, different views, and the outdoors doesn't collect dust! Whether you choose to take a trip to the gym or a jaunt around the block, either one will give you a workout. Try them both and enjoy getting in shape.

Showing Good Form

We've been walking since we were toddlers. But putting one foot in front of the other to get from point A to point B is different than using walking as a workout. This type of walking takes form and technique to prevent injuries.

To get the most out of your walking workout, make sure that you roll each hip forward to buffer the impact. Put your heel down first, roll across you foot, and then push off with your big toe. Pump your arms and take long strides to increase the benefits of your walking workouts. Pick up the pace and put pride in your stride! Remember you want to get your heart rate up and pumping.

Walking Variations

1. Speed
2. Intensity
3. Duration & Frequency
4. Interval Training

Speed and Intensity

I will refer to walking speed in terms of Slow, Moderate, Fast, and Walk-Jog. Changing your speed increases the intensity of the workout, which leads to many fitness benefits, like increased cardiovascular capacity, greater muscle strength, burning more calories, and reaching your fitness goals faster.

* **Slow:** 2.0 mph—a 30-minute mile
* **Moderate:** 3.0 mph—a 20-minute mile
* **Fast:** 4.0 mph—a 15-minute mile
* **Walk-Jog:** about 6.0 mph, depending on if you walk quickly or jog slowly

Duration and Frequency

How long you walk is the duration. If you're a novice, you'll want to walk fifteen minutes each session for your first week, then gradually increase it. Walk at a pace that gets your heart rate up, but make sure you can still talk easily. This will keep you in the heart-rate range that will give you the best workout. Fifteen minutes should cover one to two miles. By the end of eight weeks, you'll be walking sixty minutes with ease! It's true that if you put in the time, you will reap the benefits. How often you perform the workout is the frequency. The more you do the workout, the quicker your body will respond, and the faster you will reach your goals. It only makes sense! Three days a week will get you slow to moderate results and take twice as long. Five to six days a week will get you quicker results in a shorter amount of time.

Interval Training

With interval training you will vary your workouts either by intervals of rest or by changing your exercise intensity at intervals. In the walking fat burning workout, I suggest walk-jog for your intervals. By walking for two minutes then jogging for three minutes, you are doing intensity interval training. This type of training is an effective way to achieve progressive overload that develops cardio respiratory endurance while burning calories. Your heart rate or pulse will increase and decrease during interval training. I like this type of training because I don't get fatigued as quickly as I would with continuous training. It's great for first-time exercisers. You do what you can, then you ease off for a recovery period, then do it all again. Just when you think you can't take another step, it's time to recover and catch your breath!

Strength Training Basics

Believe it or not, our muscles have memories. Doing the same exercise or movement over and over again has little effect on the muscle after a while. For example, if you ask an athlete to play a completely different sport than they usually play, there's no doubt they will be sore the next day. Why? Because their muscles have become familiar with a routine. By doing different activities, they are shocking the muscles into working harder. Activities that push the muscles in different ways break down muscle fibers, leading to the soreness you feel the next day. One way to defy gravity is to keep our muscles and mind stimulated by changing it up, making our muscles work harder to fight the dreadful sagging that happens if they are neglected. "Use it or lose it" has true meaning when it comes to muscles.

Time and again, research has shown that good muscle strength helps people live healthier lives. Strong muscles can improve many areas of your life, such as decreased body fat and increased self image, not to mention helping to prevent injuries. After the age of thirty, people begin to lose muscle and bone mass. This can lead to increased risk of injuries, especially in older people. But it doesn't have to be all down hill after thirty. By incorporating exercise and healthy nutrition into your lifestyle, you can look and feel great throughout your life—no matter what your age!

As women pass fifty-five, hormonal changes, improper nutrition, and lack of exercise can cause them to develop osteoporosis, a condition in which bones become weak, porous, and easily breakable. Weight-bearing exercise and strength training increase bone density. When coupled with calcium intake and proper nutrition (see Nutrition in chapter 1), strength training can help prevent this debilitating condition.

When starting a strength training program, it's important to know how much weight or resistance you should begin with. The strength training program I have designed for the Defy Gravity Workout is based on using dumbbells or hand weights that weigh between two to ten pounds. Keep in mind, our body weight is another form of resistance that we can (and do) use on a daily basis. This is why it is so difficult for people who are extremely overweight to do much activity, because their own body weight is working against them. If you are a novice (beginner), try starting out with two or three pounds until it becomes too easy—a surefire sign that it's time to increase the weight. And don't be afraid of heavier weights giving you big muscles, ladies! We women don't have the testosterone hormone that men have to develop big muscles to show off. Remember that weights and resistance is good for us, so pick it up and pump.

In order to achieve muscular strength and endurance, you must do enough repetitions (reps) of each exercise. The heavier the weight or resistance, the fewer reps you will need to do to reach fatigue. In strength training, the group of repetitions of an exercise followed by a rest period is called a "set." In the Defy Gravity Workout, you'll be asked to do two to three sets of eight to twelve reps. How much rest do you need between sets? You usually need one to three minutes if you are lifting heavy weights. Because we are using light dumbbells for Defy Gravity, you should rest only thirty to sixty seconds between each set. If you're working only one limb at a time, then you will move continuously, switching sides. Each side rests as the other works. For instance, during a leg lift, you would do eight to twelve reps on the right leg, then do eight to twelve with the left leg, and then back to the right without any rest in between. Range of movement is the distance between the starting point of the exercise to the end, or the full motion possible in a joint. In the Defy Gravity Workout, you will count the time it takes to go through a range of motion in seconds. Slow and controlled is what we're looking for. Make each second count. Exercising slowly has more effect on your muscles.

Another question some people have is how to breathe while doing the strength training exercises. Always remember to inhale before starting the exercise and exhale during the exercise or range of motion. The most important thing is not to hold your breath.

Core and Balance Training

Every so often our industry comes out with a new buzzword. If you take any exercise classes (especially Pilates) or keep up with today's fitness magazines, you have heard that you must work your "core." Athletes have actually known about strengthening their core muscles for years.

So what exactly is the core? Like it implies, your core encompasses your deep center abdominal and lower back muscles that work to support your midsection. This important muscle group helps you balance and stabilize your body while doing certain movements. For example, if you were to reach forward to grab something that was a little out of your reach, you'd lean forward, stretch your arm, and balance on one leg. It is your core that keeps you from falling over. By strengthening your core, you improve your balance, strength, and agility.

It usually isn't until our later years that we notice a loss of balance that begins to affect our quality of life. This is why I have included exercises that require you to balance your body as you perform the exercise. This will help you strengthen your core muscles and maintain your ability to balance as you get older.

To understand why core exercises work, imagine your body as sections and limbs. Within your body you have an upper half (everything from your waist up, including your main torso, abs, back, and chest) and your lower half (your butt and legs). The muscles in your torso stabilize the rest of the sections, while your thighs help with balance. The stronger your torso, or core, is, the better control you have over your limbs. And there are no ifs, ands, or buts about how important your butt is. These two cheeks were placed there to help us stand, walk, and sit.

So how can you strengthen your core muscles to help with balance? You'll find many exercises in my Muscle Strengthening and Yoga/Pilates workouts that will help you build strength in your core. You might even find yourself balancing on one leg while doing bicep curls.

Here's a simple test to see how well you balance without trouble—stand on one leg with both arms stretched out to the sides shoulder-level. Now close your eyes and see if you can hold that position for ten seconds. If not, get ready to see major improvement with the Defy Gravity Workout!

Yoga and Pilates Basics

Yoga

Yoga is an ancient practice that refers to the union of mind, body, and soul. There are two types of yoga: Hatha, the most common yoga style, that concentrates on balance, breath, and flexibility, and Asana, a system of physical postures designed to cleanse the body, clear energy paths, and raise the level of consciousness. Besides bringing you inner peace and mental stability, yoga also improves your body's hormonal balance—an important benefit for us forty-plus women!

So how can yoga help you defy gravity? First off, we know that bone loss increases as we age. Our spine slowly degenerates over time, which can cause a hunched-over look. But weight-bearing exercises such as yoga, which uses your body weight as resistance, can prevent bone loss and build a strong skeletal system. Yoga's stretching movements also lengthen the spine and keep the flow of blood pumping strongly throughout the body.

As we've learned, stress and how we respond to it affects our bodies. It can lower our immune systems, allowing our bodies to get sick, and intensify the aging process. The deep breathing of yoga carries oxygen throughout the body and relaxes tense muscles to calm us.

The yoga poses that I have chosen in the Defy Gravity Workout are Hatha-type exercises that improve strength, flexibility, and balance, and release stress, which all help in defying gravity. In order to get the most out of yoga, it is important to focus on proper breathing, posture, and body alignment.

Breathing

You might think that it is silly to talk about breathing. After all, you're always breathing. However, it's intentional breathing during yoga that will allow you to do the positions with ease. By inhaling deeply through your nose (expanding your stomach and ribs and filling your lungs completely) and slowly exhaling through your mouth, you will increase the oxygen throughout your body. This in turn will increase blood flow in both your muscles and internal organs.

Form and Alignment

There is a reason exercise classes have mirrors. It's so you can see how your form or body alignment is during the exercise. Watching yourself in a mirror to see if your head is in line with your spine or your arms are straight is helpful in performing yoga positions correctly.

Strength and Flexibility

Each time you do the exercise you'll become a little stronger and more flexible. If you find you cannot stretch to a full pose, place your hands flat on the floor (or on the top of a yoga brick, available at most sporting goods stores). Then stretch as far as comfortable. Never stretch to the point of pain.

Pilates

Pilates is a popular type of exercise invented by a German named Joseph Pilates. He created a spring-like bed device that is known as the Reformer machine. With a series of daily exercises using pulleys and weights, Pilates instructed the Scotland Yard detectives in self-defense. After the fatal flu virus swept through Britain in 1918, Pilates concluded that his technique could also strengthen the body's immune system. This led him to develop a lifelong interest in creating exercises to aid rehabilitation following illness and injury. He continued his work by using his exercise regimen to help dancers increase their strength and agility without adding muscular bulk.

There are two ways to practice Pilates—in a group class on a mat (which is what I suggest in the Defy Gravity Workout) or private lessons using the Reformer pulley machine. Whichever one you choose, you will certainly increase your strength, flexibility, endurance, posture, coordination, and balance.

Mat Pilates is a series of calisthenic exercises done very slowly, with control and proper breathing. The breathing is similar to yoga breathing, with deep inhales through the nose, expanding your chest and belly and filling your lungs completely, then exhaling slowly through the mouth. As with yoga, breathing this way will increase the flow of oxygen throughout your body and internal organs.

Building Activity into Your Lifestyle

There are many people who will ask me, "I hate to exercise. What can I do?" There are many things you can do to include exercise into your daily life without even knowing you're doing it.

Let's begin with parking…Why drive around until you find the closest parking space? Park as far away as possible from your destination and walk! If it's the grocery store you're going into, don't let the clerk help you unload the bags of groceries into your car. I bet you didn't realize that you are doing resistance exercise by lifting and moving those bags!

At the office, or if you live in a high-rise, take the stairs, not the elevator. If you're just starting to work out, begin with walking one flight of stairs, then take the elevator the rest of the way. Once that becomes easy, take two flights of stairs, then three, and so on. Stairs are a great heart pumping activity that will keep your legs, butt, and thighs in great shape. When you're traveling, take the stairs to your room in the hotel to get in a little exercise when you're off your usual schedule.

Yard work has never been my favorite pastime, maybe because of the dirt. However, my mother, who has always been a hard-working woman, knows that yard work can be a great workout. She has an acre with a pool and does all the yard work herself. That's a lot of grass to cut, flowers to maintain, and a pool to clean. She will jump out of bed first thing in the morning and not come back into the house until late afternoon. That's a full day's work of bending, pulling, walking, kneeling, reaching, digging, and who knows what else.

Keep in mind that these types of daily activities should not be counted as your workout for the other five days, but extra things to include in your routine to burn more calories and move your body.

There are even more ways to mix fun and exercise into your daily grind. This is what I'm calling "Day Six Fun Day." This is where you incorporate a fun activity as exercise for Day six of the Defy Gravity Workout. A few examples:

✳ Playing tennis with a friend. Singles is a better workout than doubles.
(400 to 530 calories per hour)

✳ How about a bike ride with your family? Make it fun by challenging each other to race to the next stop sign. Don't forget your helmet! (480 to 750 calories per hour)

✳ If it's a winter wonderland outside, hit the slopes and ski right over that fresh pile of powder. A day of skiing will burn calories and build muscles.
(400 to 500 calories per hour)

✳ During the spring, find the perfect hiking spot, put on your hiking boots, and start climbing. Hiking is a great lower body exercise, and you'll find your heart pumping a little faster. (370 to 440 calories per hour)

✳ If your kids just got new inline skates, don your knee and elbow pads and helmet and join them for a roll around the block. Inline skating is great for the outer thighs, buns, and core muscles. (430 to 510 calories per hour)

Exercise should be fun, safe, and effective. So be creative; let your imagine run wild and let your body follow! You can make working out **fun.**

Target Heart Rate

In order to know if you are working hard enough during your workout, you need to watch your target heart rate. To determine the proper rate, subtract your age from 220. This is your MHR. Multiply this number by 65% (.65) and then 90% (.90) to find your target heart rate zone in beats per minute (bpm). This zone will give you an idea of how hard you want to work for each workout—your heart rate should reach at least 65% of your MHR and should not exceed 90% of your MHR. With the Defy Gravity Workout walking program, I'd like you to aim for about 75% to 80%.

Example: For someone forty-five years old working at a 75% intensity rate, the target heart rate is:

$$220 - 45 = 175 \qquad 175 \times .75 = 132 \text{ bpm}$$

There are a couple of ways to determine if you are reaching your target heart rate during your workout. The most obvious way is for you to take your pulse. Place your index and middle fingers on your Carotid artery (neck/throat), your Radial artery (below your thumb on your wrist), or your Temporal artery (the side of your face at brow level by your hairline. Once you feel your pulse, count the beats for six seconds, then add a zero. This will give you your approximate working heart rate.

Some people can't find their pulse or find it a nuisance to stop exercising to count. Another easy method is known as **Perceived Exertion**. This method doesn't interfere with your activity because it is based on how you're feeling during your workout (see box). One way to tell if you're working too hard is your breathing—whether you can hold a conversation during your exerciseroutine. This is a Talk Test. If you're chatting up a storm and aren't breaking a sweat this means you're not working hard enough and need to pick up the pace. If your conversation is choppy because you're gasping for breath, you're pushing too hard and need to ease off a bit.

PERCEIVED EXERTION CHART

3	Extremely Light
4	Very Light
5	Light
6	Somewhat Hard
7	Hard
8	Very Hard
9	Extremely Hard
10	Maximum Exertion

One costly way to take your heart rate is with an actual monitor that straps around your chest and a watch that reads your heart rate. These monitors can cost $100 dollars or more.

Your true maximum heart rate can be determined by your physician. Your physician will give you a stress test that is done by hooking you up to monitors while you walk on a treadmill or ride a stationary bike. You'll find once your fitness improves you're resting heart rate will decrease and you'll need to increase your intensity to reach your target heart rate.

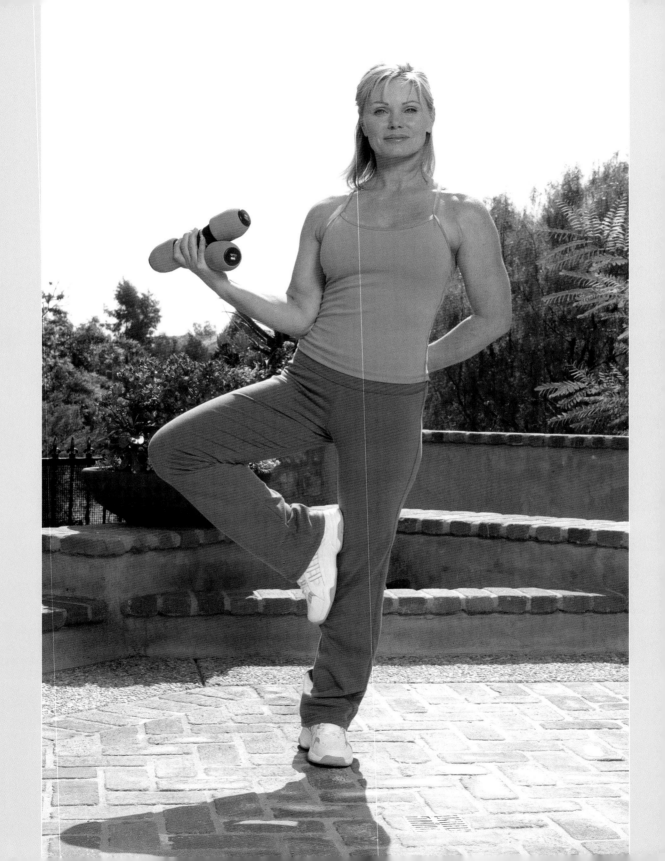

CHAPTER THREE

How to Schedule Your Workouts

We never seem to have enough time to fit all the things that we want to accomplish into one day. If time could be manufactured, bottled, and sold, that company would be the richest empire in the world! But if you learn how to manage your time, you'll always be able to fit the most important things into your day…like exercise!

The Defy Gravity Workout will take you sixty minutes, six days a week. You will be surprised how many benefits you will get out of this routine—more than you ever thought! Certainly you'll look better, feel better, and be healthier, but it's the increased energy that will shock you. It will allow you to accomplish all the other daily chores you used to just plod through.

It's important never to let your personal time with your body get pushed to the side. It's time to make time. If you're a morning person, then fit your workout in within the first two hours of rising. If that means getting up an hour earlier than your family gets up, then set that alarm clock and get moving! Joining your family for a healthy breakfast after some exercise sets the stage for a very productive day.

If afternoon is more your time to exercise, make workout time before dinner, so you feel like you've earned your meal. When I teach my evening classes, my students usually walk through the door with their minds still at the office or preoccupied with projects and tasks. But after sitting at a desk all day, they're also ready to get off their butts, move their bodies, and get their heart rates up…working off the day's ups and downs.

Adding exercise to your day is a lifestyle change, not just something you do once in a while to drop a few extra pounds. Look at your six-day schedule and see where your workouts will fit best into your life. Maybe there is someone in your family who can join you or a friend or neighbor who has been looking to get on a healthy program as well. Research from the North American Association for the Study of Obesity suggests that if you have someone who you can check in with about your progress, you are likely to lose twice as much weight as someone who doesn't. So grab someone and get moving!

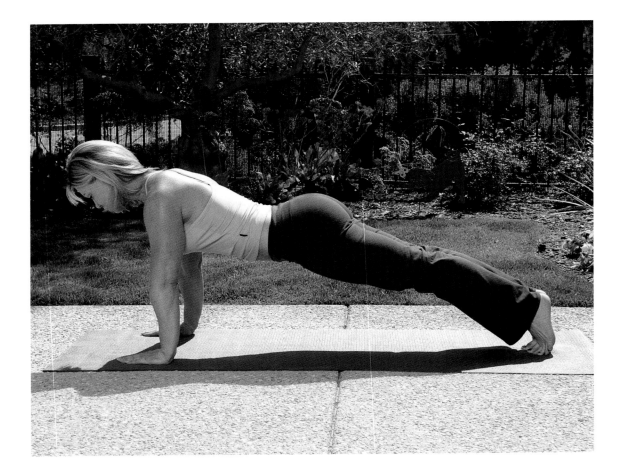

Putting Your Program Together

Those who work out to my videos wonder, "I have a Buns video, an Abs video, and a Cardio Blast video. How can I use each of the videos for the best workout?" That's a good question. Remember it this way—to put together a successful workout, you need muscle conditioning two to three times a week and cardio six days a week, with one day's rest between each workout for that particular muscle group. So to combine all of these videos, you should workout with Cardio Blast six days a week (substituting walking or jogging for one or two of those days). Then on days one and three, do the buns and abs videos. Keep in mind that you also need to work your other muscle groups, so try working your upper body on days two and four. Now you have a balanced workout program.

For the Defy Gravity Workout, it's pretty much the same thing. You want to choose one of the three walking programs (30 minutes/45 minutes/60 minutes). Whichever one you decide on will determine if you'll also do yoga/Pilates or the muscle workout. Let's say you have 60 minutes to work out Monday through Friday. Monday and Friday will be a 45-minute walking program with 15 minutes of the yoga/Pilates workout. On Tuesday and Thursday you will do the 30-minute walking program with the 30-minute muscle workout. On Wednesday and Saturday you will do the 60-minute walking program or some other choice of aerobic workout that will get your heart rate up for 60 minutes.

Another example is to do the 60-minute walking workout on Mondays and Fridays, with Tuesdays and Thursdays being a 30-minute walking with 30-minute muscle, and Saturday 45-minute walking with 15 minutes of yoga/Pilates.

But let's say you only have 15 minutes in the morning to get a quick workout in. Your best bet is to do the yoga/Pilates workout. Later in the day, do your 45-minute walking program.

I don't care how you schedule it, as long as you get into a six-day workout week with at least two days a week of the muscle workout, two days of yoga/Pilates, and five to six days of walking. Don't worry if your week changes periodically and you aren't able to follow exactly what you did last week. This is actually more beneficial. You need to keep your muscles guessing as to what's coming next, so they will work harder. You will even notice that the muscle workouts change every two weeks, increasing in intensity and duration.

In this book, I offer you an eight-week workout program, which is the time it takes to see real results. After the eight weeks, I suggest mixing in other types of activities, but keep the same days and duration of the workouts. Schedule everything to best fit into your daily routine and you'll see success!

SAMPLE WORKOUT SCHEDULE #1

- **Monday/Wednesday/Friday**

  30-minute walking workout
  30-minute muscle workout
  Stretch

- **Tuesday/Thursday**

  45-minute walking workout
  15-minute yoga/Pilates workout
  Stretch

- **Saturday**

  Fun workout (e.g. tennis)

SAMPLE WORKOUT SCHEDULE #2

- **Monday/Friday**

  60-minute walking workout
  Stretch

- **Tuesday/Thursday**

  30-minute walking workout
  30-minute muscle workout
  Stretch

- **Wednesday**

  45-minute walking workout
  15-minute yoga/Pilates workout
  Stretch

- **Saturday**

  Fun workout (e.g. bike riding)

SAMPLE WORKOUT SCHEDULE #3

- **Monday**

  15-minute yoga/Pilates workout A.M.
  45-minute walking workout P.M.

- **Tuesday**

  60-minute walking workout

- **Wednesday**

  30-minute muscle workout A.M.
  30-minute walking workout P.M.

- **Thursday**

  15-minute yoga/Pilates workout A.M.
  45-minute walking workout P.M.

- **Friday**

  Fun workout (e.g. Swimming 60 minutes)

- **Saturday**

  30-minute muscle workout
  30-minute walking workout

TIGHT ON TIME WORKOUT

This workout should be done only if you cannot get to your Defy Gravity Workouts. Once in a while, we have a day that will only allow us ten free minutes, and I always say ten minutes toward your personal health is better than none!

If you want more information on tight-on-time workouts, check out my website, **www.tamileeweb.com**, or **www.naturaljourneys.com**.

Do all of these exercises, then repeat from the beginning as many times as your tight-on-time schedule allows:

- Push-ups   20
- Crunches   25
- Tricep dips   20
- Step Ups   20 each leg

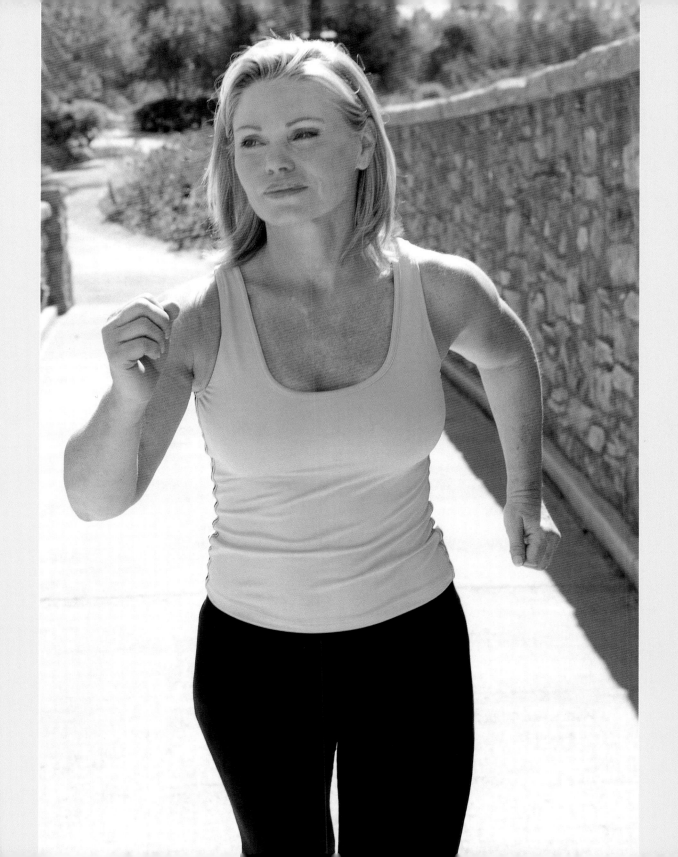

Stretches

Part of being healthy and fit is to have flexibility. Having a range of motion without pain and discomfort is important to our joints A good stretching program also helps reduce injuries. When we exercise, our muscles get tight due to their contractions during movement. By stretching and relaxing your muscles after a workout, you can release the tightness and any pressure the joints might have felt as a result.

There are many types of stretching, but the one I'm going to recommend is **Static Stretching.** This is where the muscle is gradually stretched to the point of tightness (not pain) and held for ten to thirty seconds while breathing deeply. Of course, the longer you hold the stretch, the greater the benefits.

One of the best things I love about stretching is how I feel an inch taller and ten pounds lighter afterwards. For more stretching and relaxation, please check out my two stretch videos/DVDs: *Total Body Stretch* shows you three ten-minute stretching routines done standing, sitting, or lying on the floor, and *Stretch and Relaxation* gives you thirty minutes of yoga-type stretches. It also includes a five-minute visual relaxation mediation segment. (You can find these videos at **www.tamileewebb.com**.)

It is best to warm up with a light physical activity (like walking or jogging for five minutes) before stretching. Please make sure you stretch after each workout. Hold each stretch for ten to thirty seconds, and breathe through the stretch.

✳ Standing Calves

1. Step forward with your left leg into a slight lunge. Press the heel of your right foot down into the ground. Lower yourself more into the lunge for a deeper stretch. Make sure the knee of your front leg stays at a right angle to your ankle.

2. One of my favorite stretches for the calves is to stand on the edge of a step, drop one heel off of the step and press through your heel with a slightly bent knee. Switch legs.

Stretches: calf, heel

✳ Standing Quads

1. Hold a chair or wall to help you balance, grab one foot and pull it toward your rear end, keeping your knee pointed toward the ground.

2. Press your hips forward and ease your foot toward your butt. Keep your knees together. Repeat on your other leg.

Stretches: quadriceps (front of thigh)

✳ Standing Hamstrings

1. Standing in front of a step or chair, raise your right leg up and rest it on the step/chair. Only lift as high as you can comfortably. Straighten your right leg as you bend your torso slightly forward from the hips, stretching long over your leg. Repeat on your left leg.

Stretches: hamstrings (back of thigh)

✳ Inner Thigh Side Lunge

1. Stand with your feet wide apart, then shift your hips to the right side, bending your right knee. Keep your knee open, hands on your thighs, and lower your torso forward gently.

2. Hold the stretch then repeat on the left side. Do not allow your knee to go past your foot.

Stretches: adductors (inner thighs)

✳ Standing Upper Back

1. Stand with both arms stretched out in from of your chest, hands interlocked. Drop your chin to your chest and round your upper back and shoulders as you reach your hands forward.

Stretches: upper back

✳ Standing Hip Flexor

1. Step your right leg forward into a lunge position. With your left leg stretched behind you, tuck your butt under, contract your abdominal muscles, and press your hips forward. Repeat on the other leg.

Stretches: hip flexors

✳ Overhead Side Stretch

1. Stand with both arms raised over your head, fingers interlocked. Stretch up as high as you can, lifting through your upper side muscles. Try to stretch up through your hands without lifting your shoulders toward your ears.

2. Lean to your right and hold, then to the left and hold.

Stretches: lattisumius dorsi (side of torso)

✳ Standing Chest Stretch

1. Stand with your feet shoulder-width apart, your knees slightly bent, and your toes pointing forward. Clasp your hands behind your back. Slowly straighten your arms and then lift them up behind your back.

Stretches: pectorals (chest)

✳ Shin Stretch

1. While standing, place your right foot behind you with top of the foot pressed against the floor. Press your foot into the floor to feel a stretch in your shin.

2. If you're near a step or ledge, place your toes on the ledge and press into it while your heel drop. Repeat stretch on the left shin.

Stretches: shin

DON'T FORGET...

- Stretch before and after your workout

- If you consider yourself a novice (someone who does little to no exercise), please refer to the asterisk (*) within each workout week.

- The walking workouts require a watch with a second hand to time yourself with the intervals. Include one of these walking workouts four to five days a week.

- If it's a day you're including the muscle strengthening workout, choose the 30-minute walking program. On a day you're including the yoga/Pilates workout, do the 45-minute walking program. Days you do not include one of the other programs, do the 60-minute walking program.

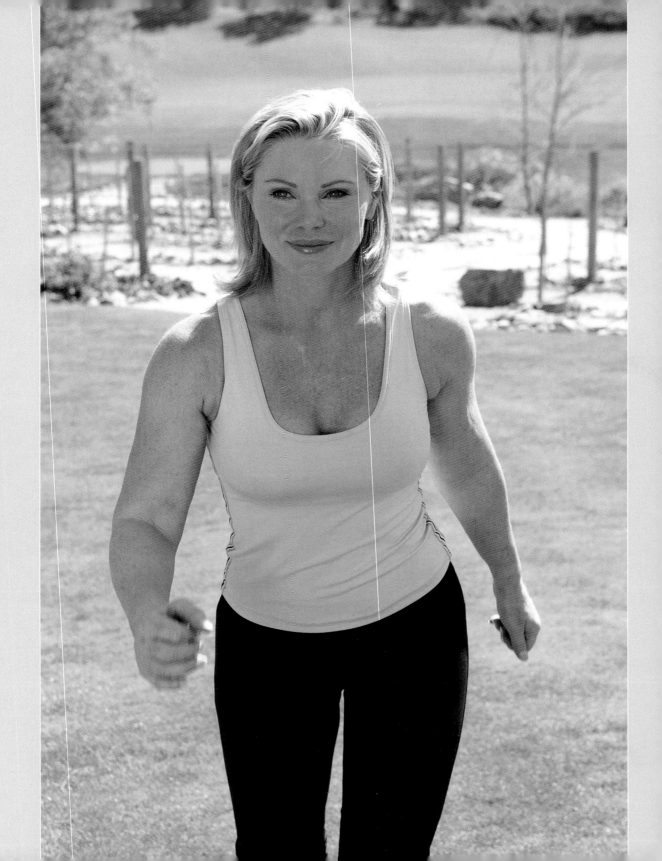

CHAPTER FOUR

Walking Routines

Because walking is the easiest exercise in the world, many of us don't actually create a program to use when we head out the door. Unfortunately, that often turns our walk into a stroll. You need to be conscious of how intensely you are walking to make sure this is a workout, not a "walk in the park" (pardon the pun). So, follow these programs. As you get used to walking with a purpose, you'll be able to create your own programs that allow you to vary your intensities and workout times, so you'll see results.

STREET WALK

30-Minute Walking
Plus Strength Workout

Moderate walk, 10 minutes

Fast walk 30 seconds, alternated
 with 60-second moderate walk

Do 10 sets

• Check heart rate

Moderate to slow walk, 5 to 10 minutes

* Try walking for 15 minutes or longer

Option:

Moderate walk, 5 minutes

Walk/jog, 3 minutes, alternated
 with 2-minute moderate walk

Do 4 sets

• Check heart rate

Moderate walk, 5 minutes

45-Minute Walking
Plus Yoga/Pilates Workout

Moderate walk, 10 minutes

Fast walk, 3 minutes, alternated with
 2-minute moderate walk

Do 5 sets

• Check heart rate

Moderate walk, 10 minutes

* Try walking for 30 minutes or longer

60-Minute Walking

Moderate walk, 10 minutes

Walk/jog, 3 minutes, alternated with
 2-minute moderate walk

Do 4 sets

• Check heart rate

Moderate walk, 5 minutes

Walk/jog, 3 minutes, alternated with
 2-minute moderate walk

Do 4 sets

Moderate walk, 5 minutes

* Try walking for 45 minutes or longer

TREADMILL WALK

30-Minute Walking
Plus Strength Workout

Moderate walk, flat (no incline),
 10 minutes

Fast walk, flat, 15 minutes

• Check heart rate

Moderate to slow walk, 5 minutes

Option:

Moderate walk, 5 minutes

Walk/jog, 3 minutes, alternated with
 2-minute moderate walk

Do 4 sets

• Check heart rate

Moderate walk, 5 minutes

45-Minute Walking
Plus Yoga/Pilates Workout

Moderate walk, flat (no incline),
 5 minutes

Fast walk at incline level one, 5 minutes

Walk/jog, flat, 3 minutes, alternated
 with walk at incline level one for
 2 minutes

Do 5 sets

• Check heart rate

Fast walk, flat, 5 minutes

Moderate to slow walk, flat, 5 minutes

60-Minute Walking

Moderate walk flat, 5 minutes

Moderate to fast walk at incline level `
 two, 5 minutes

Walk/jog, flat, 3 minutes, alternated
 with 2-minute fast walk

Do 4 sets

• Check heart rate

Moderate to fast walk 5 minutes at
 incline level two

Walk/jog, flat, 3 minutes, alternated
 with 2-minute fast walk

Do 4 sets

Moderate to slow walk flat, 5 minutes

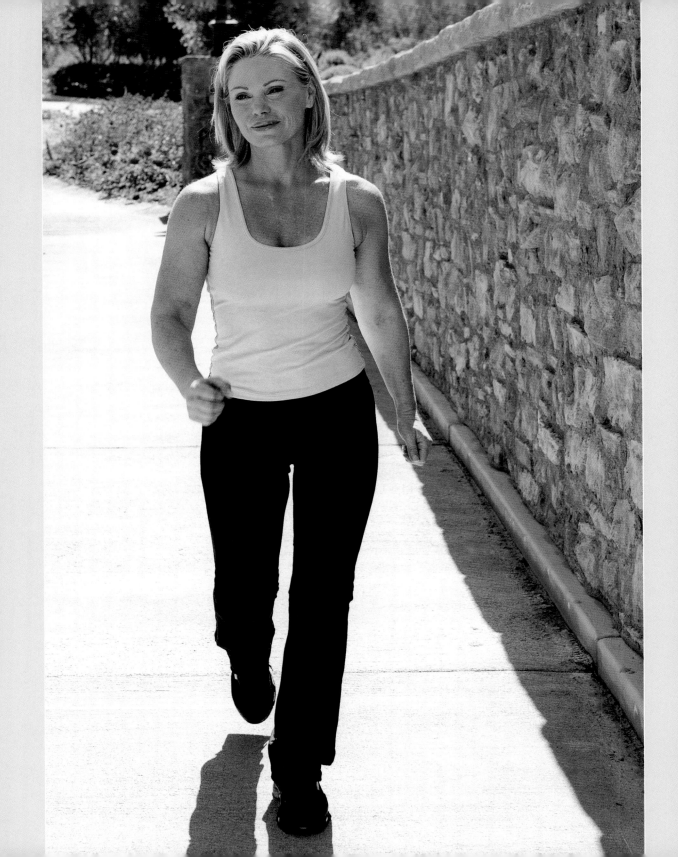

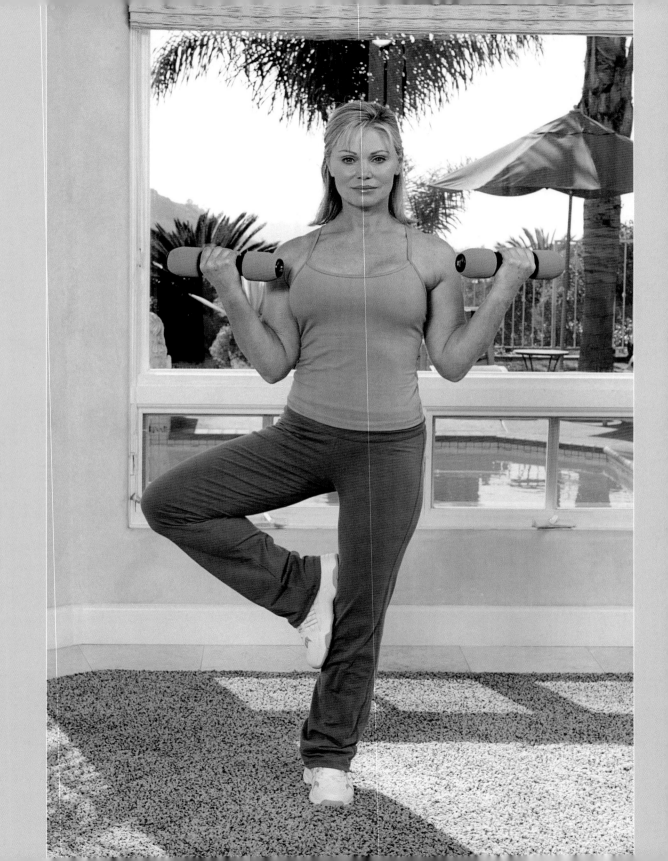

Strength Training Exercises

After just two weeks on this program you are going to fall in love with your dumbbells—because nothing changes the shape of your body more than strength training. It re-shapes and shrinks your body in amazing ways. The most important thing to remember about strength-training is that your muscle should feel fatigued by the end of each set or group of repetitions. Also, move slowly and deliberately—don't let momentum move the weight. Finally, try to stretch each muscle a little bit after doing a move—studies show that stretching helps build muscle faster.

Weeks One and Two

Week one, do two sets of ten reps of each exercise.
Week two, do three sets of ten reps of each exercise.

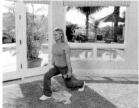 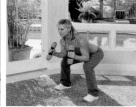 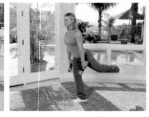 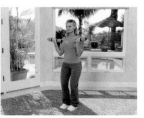

1. **Alternating Forward Lunges** (page 58)

2. **Alternating Side Squats** (page 60)

3. **Hip Extension/ Kick Backs** (page 62)

4. **Bicep Curls** (page 59)

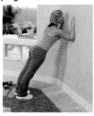 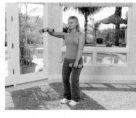 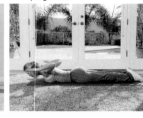 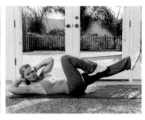

5. **Tricep Wall Push-ups** (page 64)

6. **Alternating Front Shoulder Raises** (page 65)

7. **Prone Torso Lift with Arms Raised** (page 66)

8. **Abdominal Bicycles** (page 68)

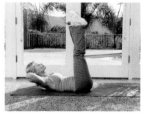

9. **Vertical Abdominal Lifts** (page 70)

Weeks Three and Four

Week three, do two sets of ten reps of each exercise.
Week four, do three sets of ten reps of each exercise.

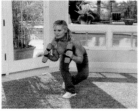

1. One-Legged Squats (page 67)

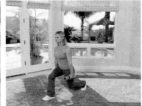

2. Traveling Lunges (page 72)

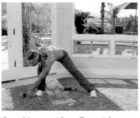

3. Alternating Reaching Side Lunges (page 74)

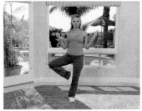

4. One-Legged Bicep Curls (page 76)

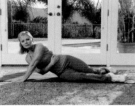

5. Side One-Arm Tricep Push-ups (page 77)

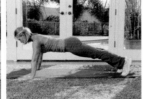

6. Push-ups (page 78)

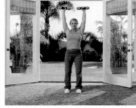

7. Overhead Shoulder Press (page 80)

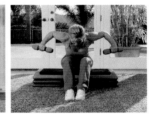

8. Bent Over Seated Rows (page 81)

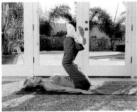

9. Reverse Abdominal Crunch (page 82)

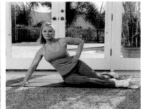

10. Side Abdominal Crunch (page 83)

Weeks Five and Six

Week five, do two sets of ten reps of each exercise.
Week six, do three sets of ten reps of each exercise.

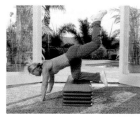 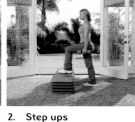 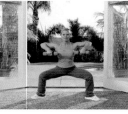 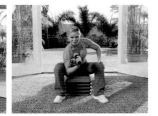

1. 90-degree Kick Backs (page 84)
2. Step ups (page 86)
3. Plié Squats (page 88)
4. Concentration Bicep Curls (page 89)

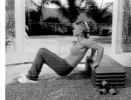 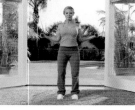 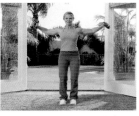

5. Squat, Bicep Curl, and Overhead Press (page 90)
6. Tricep Dips (page 92)
7. External Rotation (page 93)
8. Lateral Shoulder Raises (page 94)

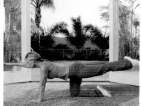 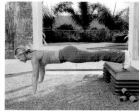 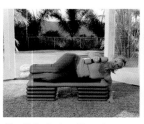 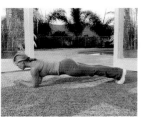

9. Balance Hands/ Knees (Bird Dog) (page 95)
10. Push-ups with Feet on Step (page 96)
11. Side-Lying One-Arm Shoulder Lift (page 98)
12. Plank (page 100)

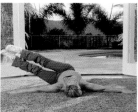 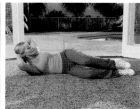

13. Abdominal Arcs (page 102)
14. Side-Lying Obliques (page 104)

Weeks Seven and Eight

Week seven, do two sets of ten reps of each exercise.
Week eight, do three sets of ten reps of each exercise.

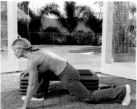

1. Runner's Lunge
   (page 106)

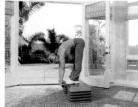

2. Dead Lifts
   (page 108)

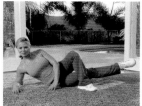

3. Side Leg Lifts on Floor
   (page 110)

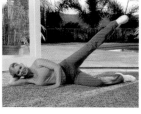

4. One-Legged Inner
   Thigh Lifts on Floor
   (page 112)

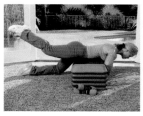

5. Prone Single Leg Lifts
   (page 114)

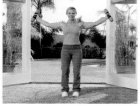

6. Marquee Shoulder Lift
   (page 116)

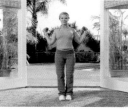

7. "W" Bicep Curl
   (page 118)

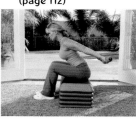

8. Rear Shoulder Raises
   (page 119)

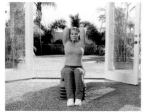

9. Overhead Tricep
   Extension (page 120)

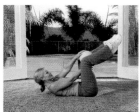

10. Pass the Ball
    Abdominal Crunch
    (page 122)

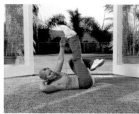

11. Diagonal Arm and
    Leg Lift (page 124)

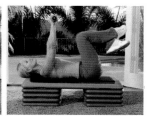

12. Chest Press on Step
    (page 126)

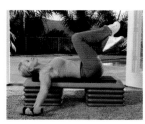

13. Chest Flies on Step
    (page 127)

The Exercises...

Alternating Forward Lunges

Works: Legs, thighs, buns, and core

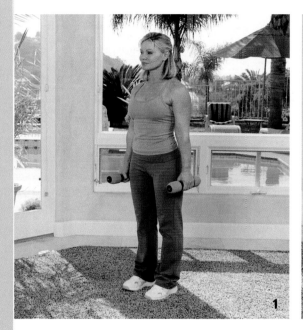

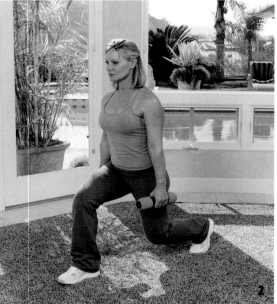

1. Stand with your feet shoulder-width apart, dumbbells in each hand. Step forward with your right leg and lunge down. Do not allow your front knee to go past your fcot.

2. Contract your abdominal muscles and push yourself back to the starting position by pressing through your right heel.

3. Repeat on your left leg. keep your shoulders down, head up, and back straight.

Bicep Curls

Works: Front of upper arm (bicep)

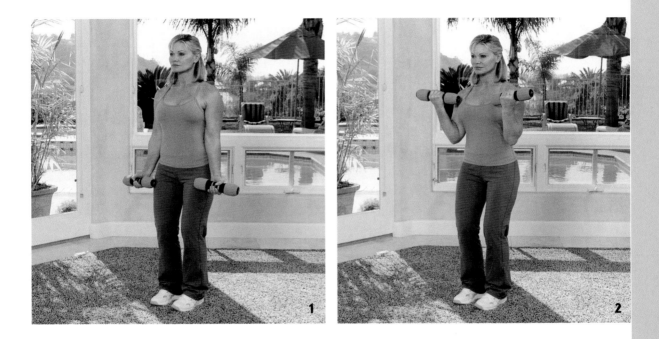

1. Stand with your weights in your hands, arms down by your side.

2. Curl both hands/weights up toward your chest for four slow counts.

3. Release the curl slowly back toward the floor for four counts. Repeat.

Alternating Side Squats

Works: Legs, thighs, buns, and core

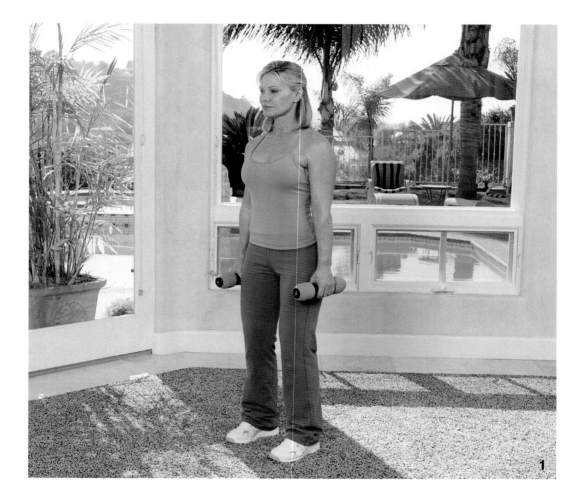

TAMILEE WEBB'S DEFY GRAVITY WORKOUT

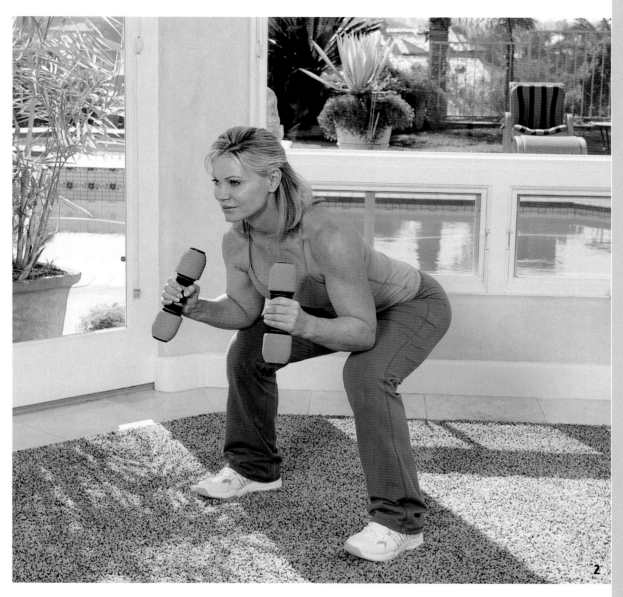

2

1. Stand with your feet shoulder-width apart, weights in each hand.

2. Step out to the right side and squat, bringing your body down to a 45- to 90-degree angle. Push off your right foot to return to the starting position.

3. Repeat on the left side. Do not allow your knees to go past your feet.

61

Hip Extension/ Kick Backs

Works: Buns and thighs

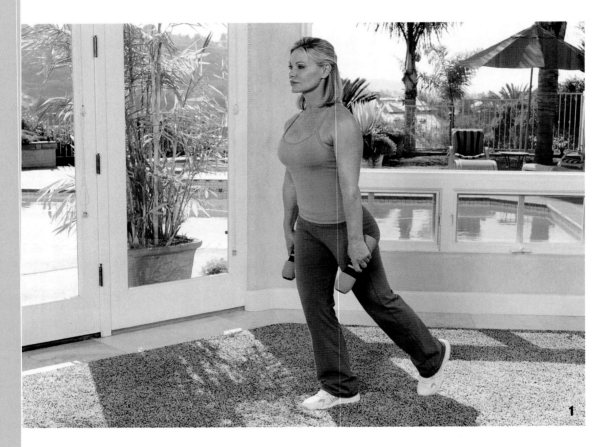

1. Stand with a weight in each hand and your legs slightly flexed at your knees and hips.

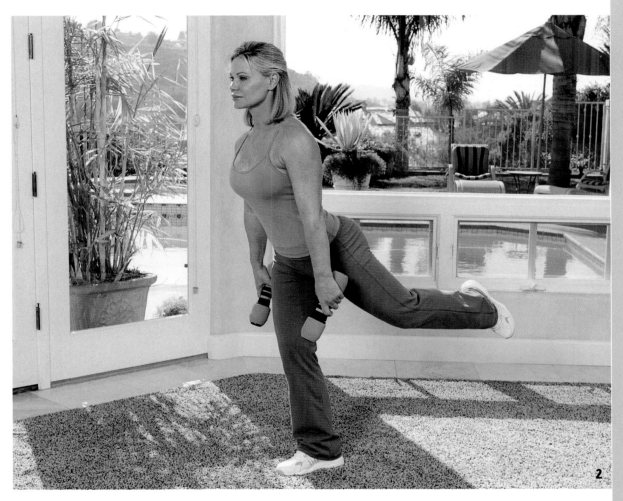

2. Lift and extend your left leg back. Contract your abdominal muscles and butt. Repeat with your right leg, keeping your hips facing forward.

Tricep Wall Push-Ups

Works: Back of upper arm (tricep) and chest (pectorals)

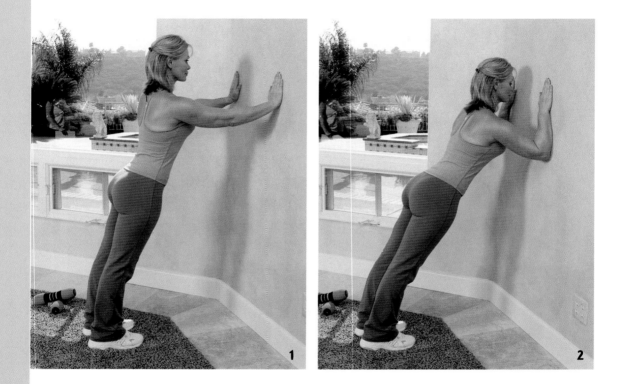

1. Stand two to three feet away from a wall and place your hands slightly wider than your shoulders on the wall.

2. Start with straight arms, inhale, then slowly exhale as you bend your arms to lower yourself toward the wall in four counts.

Once your elbows are at a 90-degree angle, inhale. Exhale and press yourself back to starting position in four counts.

3. Remember to keep your abdominal muscles pulled in to help support your back—pull your belly button to your spine. Repeat.

Alternating Front Shoulder Raises

Works: Shoulders, arms, and upper back

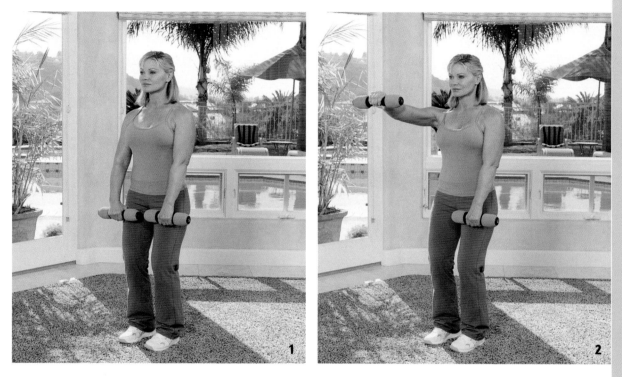

1. Stand with your feet shoulder-width apart, knees slightly bent, dumbbells in each hand.

2. Inhale, then exhale as you slowly lift your right arm up to shoulder height, palm facing down, for two counts. Keep your elbow slightly bent and your abdominal muscles pulled in.

3. Slowly return to the starting position and repeat on your left arm.

Prone Torso Lift with Arms Raised

Works: Lower and upper back, back of shoulders, and abdominals

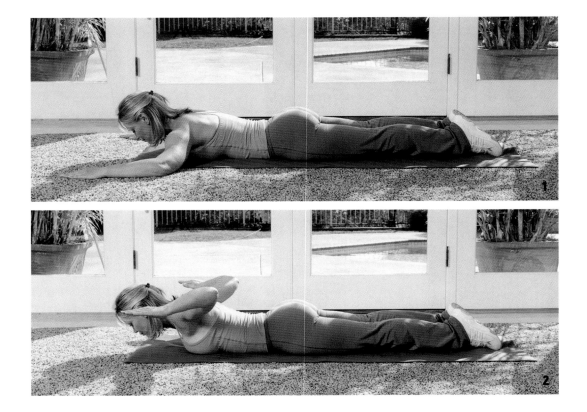

1. Lie face down on the floor, arms bent at shoulder level. Inhale then, as you exhale, lift your torso, arms, and head off of the floor.

2. Keep your butt and abdominal muscles contracted as you lift.

3. Slowly return to the starting position and repeat.

One-Legged Squats

Works: Buns, thighs, and biceps

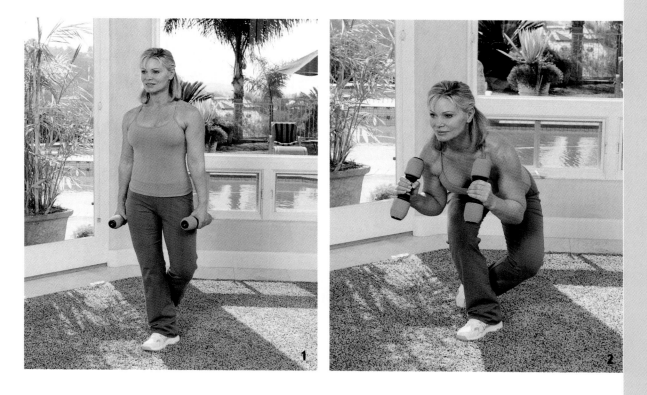

1. Stand with your weights in your hands, arms down by your side.

2. Curl both hands/weights up toward your chest for four slow counts.

3. Release the curl slowly back toward the floor for four counts. Repeat.

Abdominal Bicycles

Works: Abdominals/core

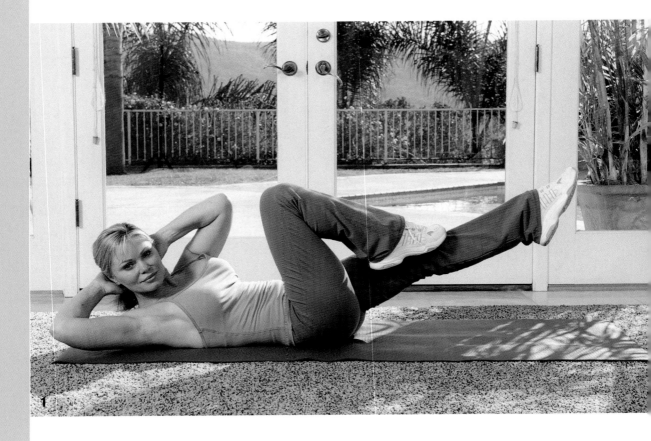

1. Lie on your back with your knees bent above your hips and hands behind your head. Extend your left leg out parallel with the floor while you rotate your torso and bring your left shoulder and elbow across to your right knee.

2. Smoothly switch sides. Keep your head in line with your spine, alternating from one side to the other.

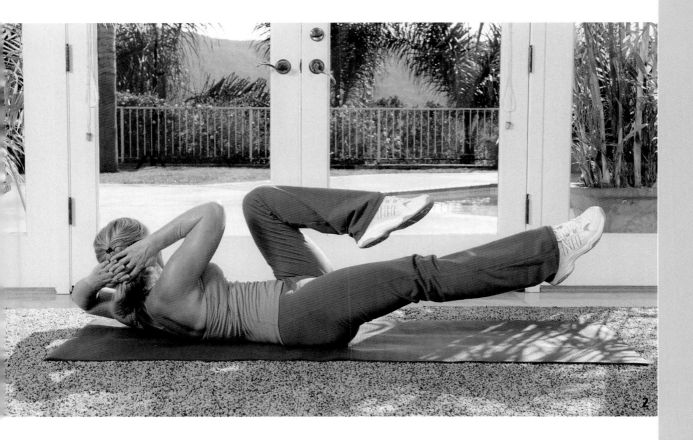

Vertical
Abdominal Lifts

Works: Abdominals/core

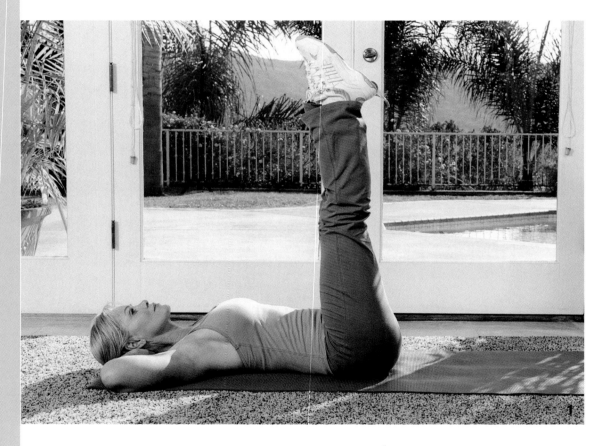

1. Lie on your back with both legs pointed straight up to the ceiling, both hands behind your head for support.

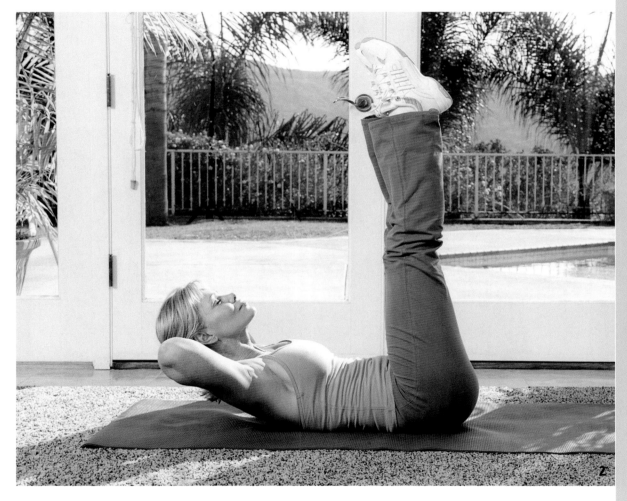

2. Raise your torso up toward your extended legs for two counts, keeping your head in line with your spine. Do not pull on your head with your hands.

3. Return to the starting position and repeat.

Traveling Lunges

Works: Buns, back of upper thigh, hamstrings, and thigh

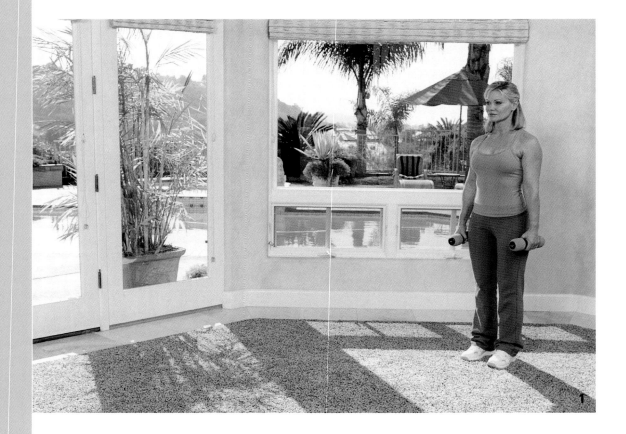

TAMILEE WEBB'S DEFY GRAVITY WORKOUT

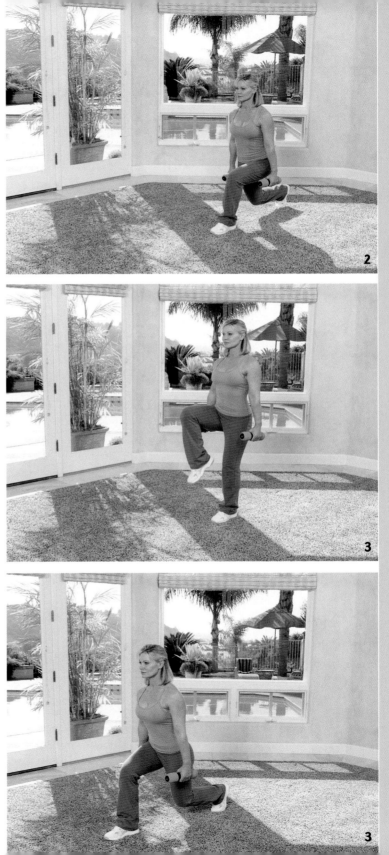

1. Stand with your hands on your waist or with a weight in each hand.

2. Step forward with your left leg and lunge. Do not allow your knee to go past your foot.

3. Continue moving forward by bringing your right knee up to waist level, then step forward into a right lunge.

4. Repeat with your left leg.

Alternating Reaching Side Lunges

Works: Buns, inner thighs, back of upper thigh, and front thigh

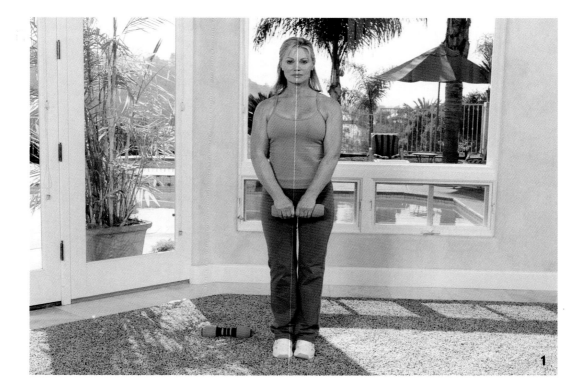

1

1. Stand with your feet together and hold one weight in front of you.

2. Step out to the right side and lunge into your right leg while reaching with your left arm and weight to the floor in front of your right foot. Your right arm can rest on your waist.

3. Push off from your right foot and return to the starting position. Repeat on the left side; continue to alternate sides.

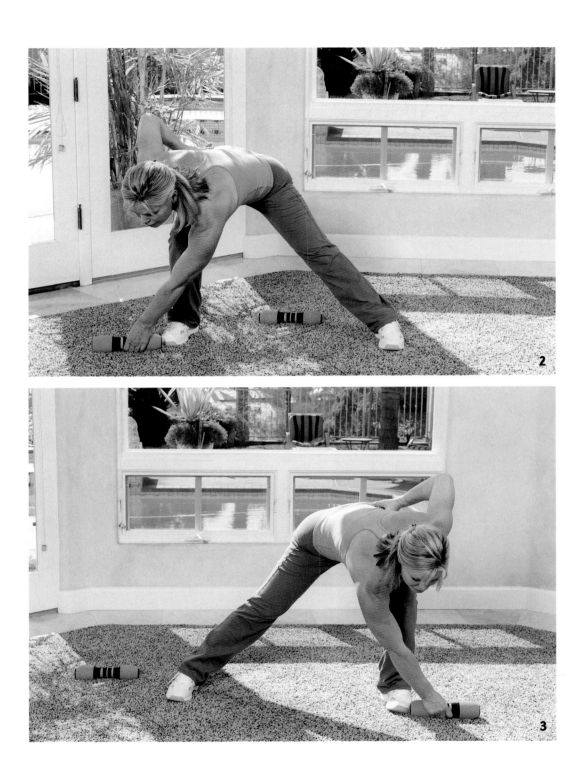

One-Legged Bicep Curls

Works: Core and upper arm (bicep)

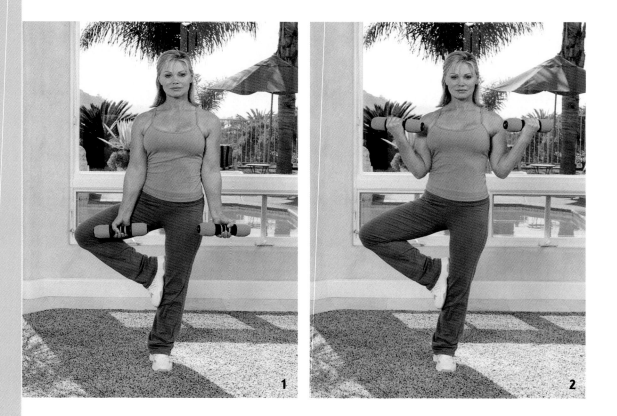

1. Stand on your left leg and place your right foot on the inside of your left thigh with your bent knee pointing toward the outside. Hold a weight in each hand—the one in your right hand should be inside your thigh.

2. Curl your arms up toward your shoulders while balancing on your left leg. Four counts up and four counts down.

3. Repeat on your right leg.

Side One-Arm Tricep Push-Ups

Works: Back of upper arm (tricep) and shoulder

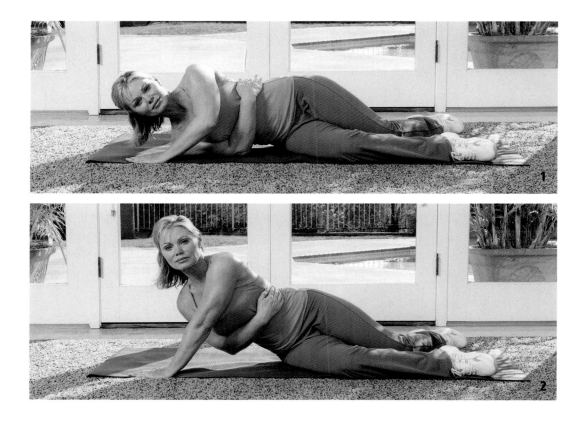

1. Lie on the floor on your right side, knees bent, with your right arm wrapped around your torso and your left hand flat in front on your right shoulder.

2. Press your torso up off the floor by straightening your left arm. Slowly return down to the starting position and repeat.

3. Repeat on your left side.

   VARIATION: If you are a novice or find this too difficult, extend your right arm out from your shoulder, palm on the floor. Press your torso up off the floor, then lower back down.

Push-Ups

Works: Chest, shoulders, and abdominals

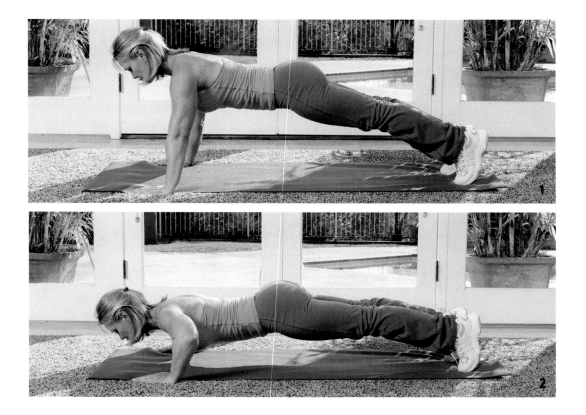

1. Face the floor on all fours, then place your hands slightly wider than your shoulders. Extend your legs straight out behind you and lift up on your toes. Pull in your abdominal muscles and straighten your arms.

2. Slowly lower your body down toward the floor for two counts then back up for two counts. It's important to keep your abdominals pulled in and your head in line with your spine. Repeat.

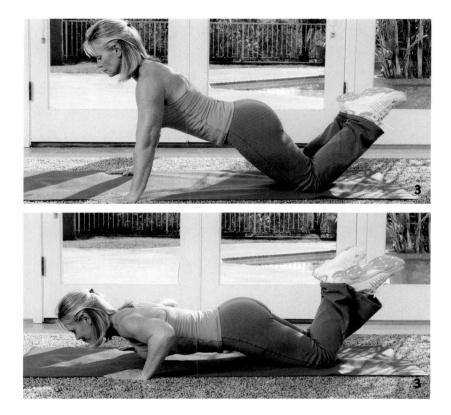

VARIATION: If you are a novice or find this too difficult, put both knees on the floor instead of straight legs to do the push up. It is still important to keep your body straight. Don't bend at the waist—lower your whole body down to the floor, not just your chest.

Overhead Shoulder Press

Works: Shoulders

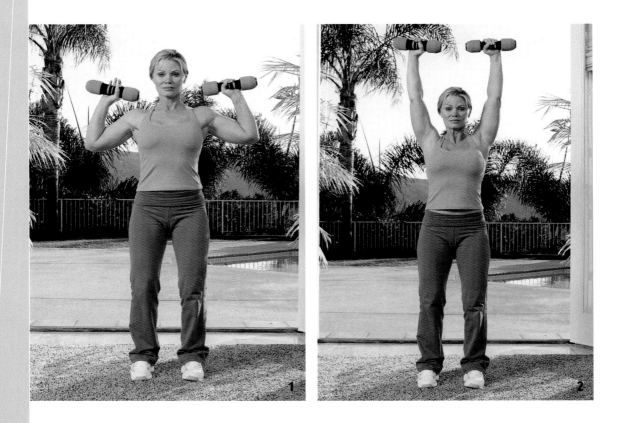

1. Stand either on the floor or a step, with a weight in each hand next to your shoulders, palms facing front.

2. Contract your abdominal muscles to balance your body and press both arms straight up over your head for four counts.

3. Slowly return to the starting position for four counts and repeat.

Bent Over Seated Rows

Works: Upper back and rear shoulders (deltoids)

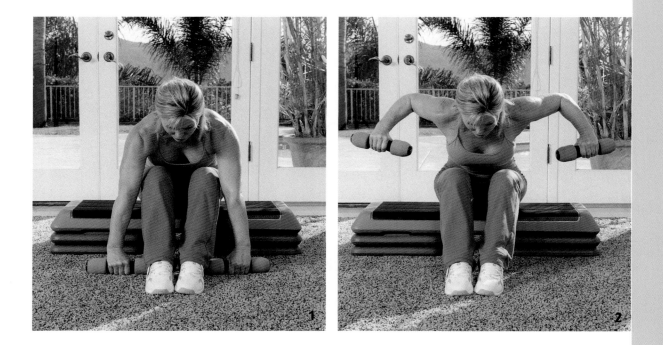

1. Sit on a step or chair with dumbbells in each hand. Lean slightly forward, keeping your back straight, and extend your arms toward the floor on either side of your legs.

2. Slowly bring your elbows back behind your shoulders and squeeze your shoulder blades together. Keep your head in line with your spine and your shoulders pressed away from your ears, pull your abdominal muscles in, and breathe.

3. Release and repeat.

Reverse Abdominal Crunch

Works: Abdominals

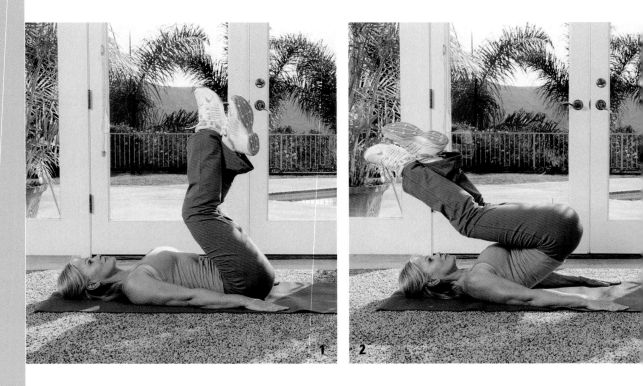

1. Lie on your back with your legs above your hips, knees bent, and your arms straight down by your side, palms down.

2. Slowly contract your abdominal muscles while pulling your knees up toward your shoulders. Slowly return to the starting position and repeat.

Side Abdominal Crunch

Works: Abdominals and obliques (side of torso)

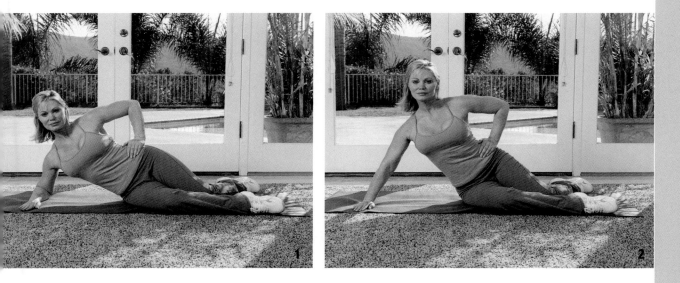

1. Lie on your right side on the floor with your knees bent. Prop yourself up on your right forearm and place your left hand on your hip.

2. Use your obliques (side abdominal muscles) to lift your body up straight.

3. Release and repeat for one set of reps, then repeat on the other side.

I like to call these the Jane Fonda; remember she used to do these all the time?

90-Degree
Kick Backs

Works: Buns and hamstrings (back of upper thigh)

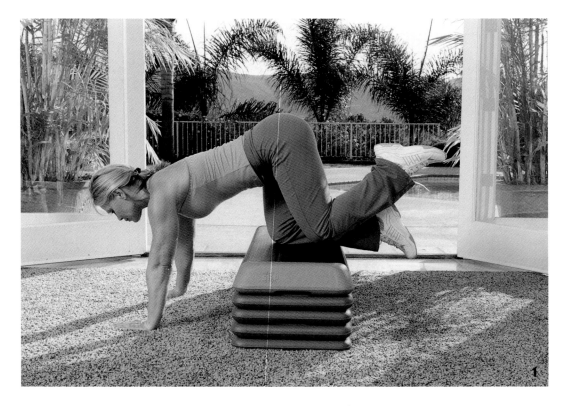

1. Kneel on a step or the seat of a
chair with your hands braced on
the floor under your shoulders.
Your hips and knees need to be
at a 45- to 90-degree angle to
one another.

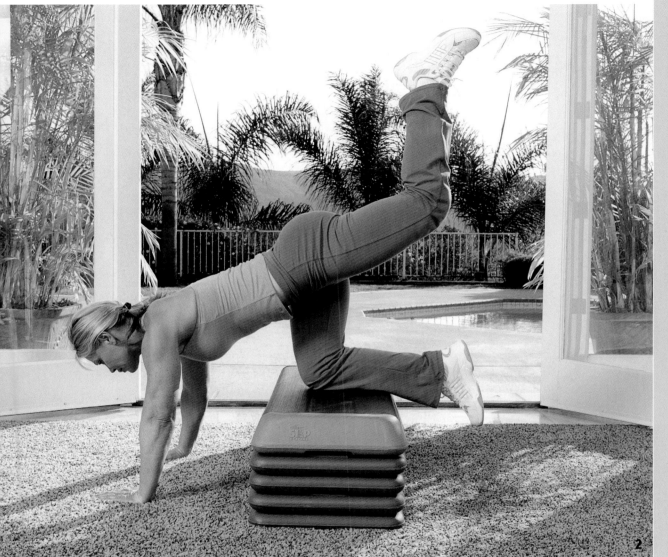

2

2. Lift your left leg with your knee bent and extend it backwards and up as if you were kicking backwards. Keep your knee at a 90-degree angle; don't straighten your leg.

3. Release and repeat for one set of reps. Repeat on the other leg. Keep your abdominal muscles pulled in and your hips stationary.

Step Ups

Works: Buns, thighs, and hamstrings (back of upper thigh)

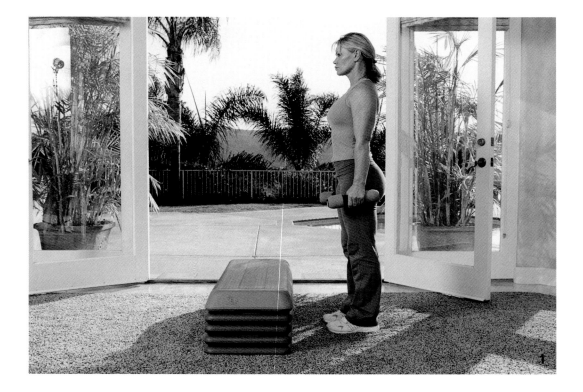

1. Stand in front of a step or sturdy stool with weights in each hand.

2. Place your left foot on the step and lift your body up and bring your right foot up onto the step. Step down with your left foot and then right.

3. Repeat for one set of reps and then switch legs.

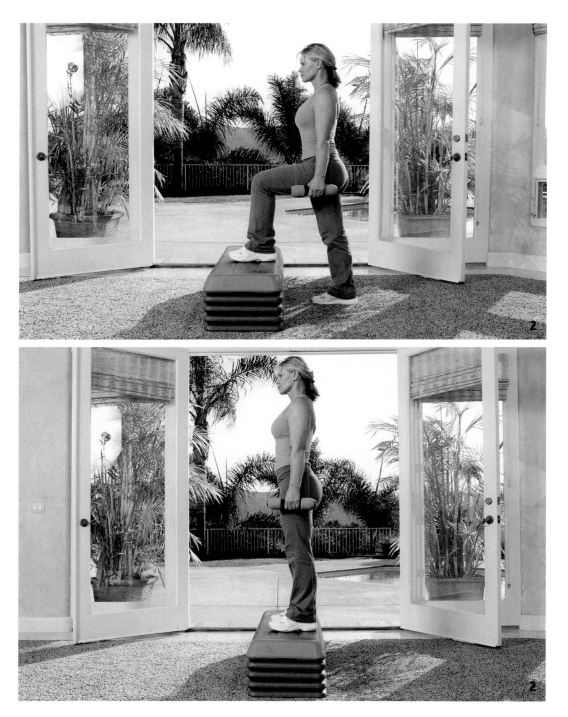

This can be done without weights.

Plié Squats

Works: Inner thigh, quads (upper thigh), and buns

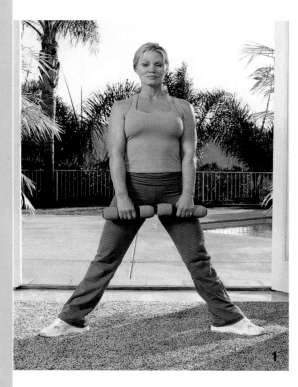
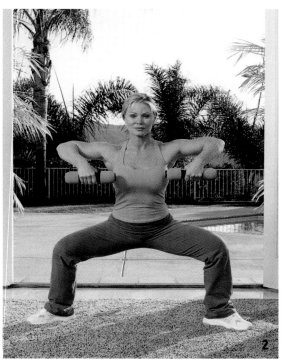

1. Stand with your feet wide apart, toes pointed out. Hold your weights in front of your hips.

2. Keeping your knees directly in line with your feet, lower your body down for four counts until your knees reach a 90-degree angle. Keep your back straight and hips tucked under. As you squat, bend your elbows and lift your weights to chest height, keeping your neck long and shoulders down.

3. Return to starting position and repeat.

Concentration Bicep Curls

Works: Bicep (upper arm)

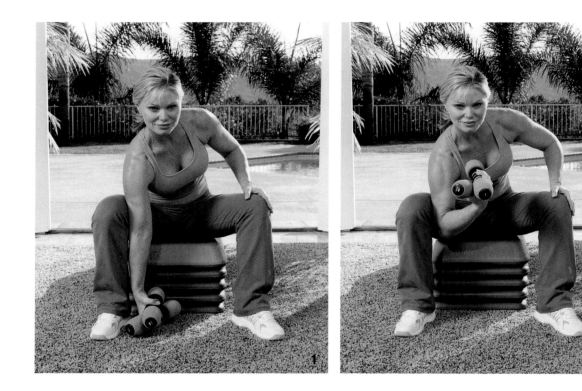

1. Sit on a step or chair with one weight in your right hand. Press your right arm into the inside of your right thigh for support. Brace your left hand on your left thigh.

2. Slowly curl your right hand in and up toward your right shoulder. Curl for four counts and release slowly for four counts.

3. Repeat for one set of reps and then switch to your left arm. Remember to keep your shoulders down, chest up, and torso steady.

Combination Squat, Bicep Curl, and Overhead Press

Works: Buns, thighs, biceps, and shoulders

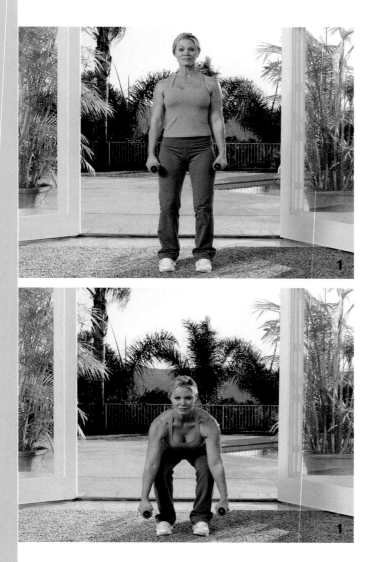

1. Stand with dumbbells in each hand, feet shoulder-width apart, and your arms down by your side. Slowly squat until your knees are at a 45- to 90-degree angle for a count of one and back up to the starting position on another count of one. You will count to eight for the whole sequence; this move is counts one and two.

2. Curl both arms up to your chest, lower them back down, then curl them up again. You are doing one and a half curls, counting three, four, and five.

3. From the top of the last bicep curl, rotate your wrists inward and press both arms up and over your head for count six, return them down to shoulder height on seven, and release to the starting position on count eight. Repeat.

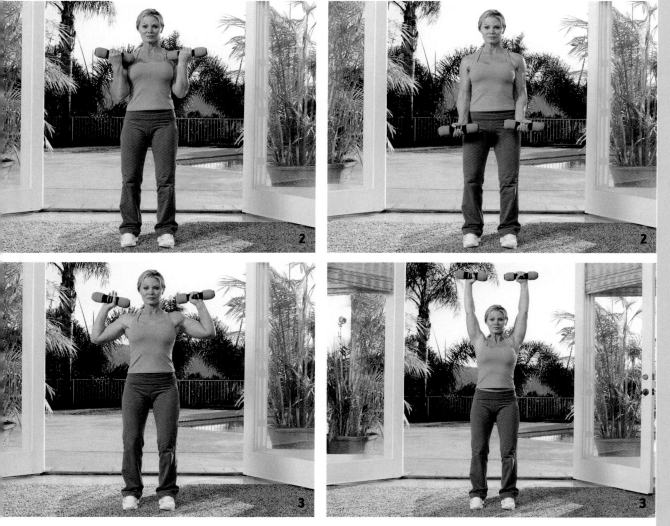

Tricep Dips

Works: Triceps (back of upper arm)

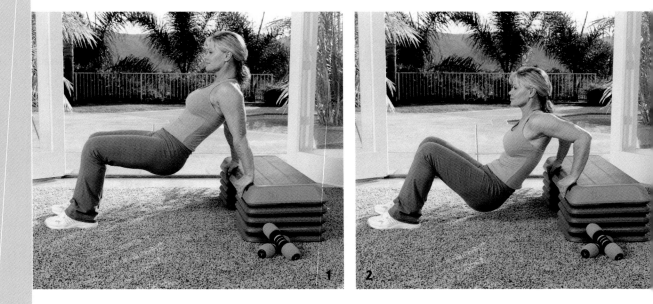

1. Sit on a step or chair, placing both hands on the edge of the step/chair, with your fingers off the edge. Slide your body off the step, keeping your arms straight.

2. Slowly lower your body down by bending your elbows as far as you can comfortably, then press your body back up by straightening your arms. Keep your shoulders pressed down away from your ears.

3. Repeat.

External Rotation

Works: Shoulders and upper back, some biceps

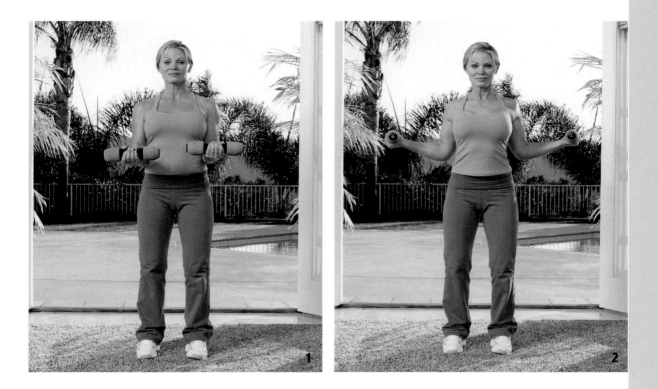

1. Stand with dumbbells in both hands and bend your arms up to a 90-degree angle with your palms up and out in front of your torso. Keep your elbows close to your body.

2. Press both arms outward, rotating from your shoulders to squeeze your shoulder blades together and press your chest forward.

3. Release and repeat.

Lateral Shoulder Raises

Works: Shoulders

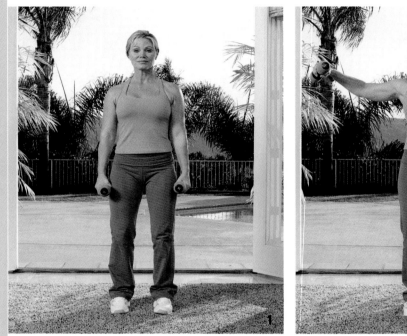
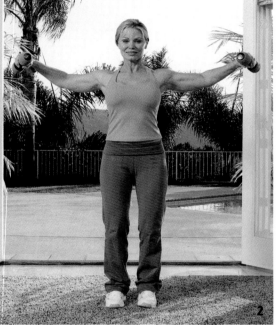

1. Stand with dumbbells in each hand and your arms at your sides.

2. Slowly lift both arms out and up to shoulder level for four counts. Keep your elbows slightly bent, palms facing down, and your abdominal muscles contracted.

3. Release for four counts and repeat.

Balance Hands/Knees (Bird Dog)

Works: Core, abdominals, and back

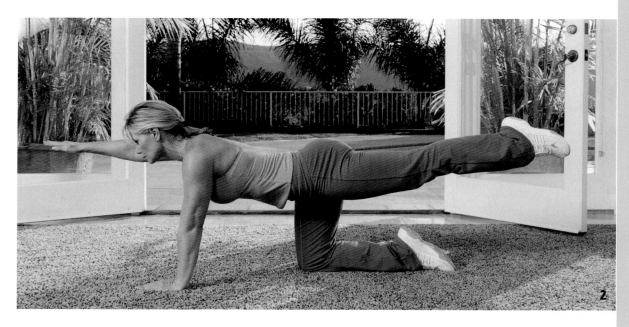

1. Kneel on the floor on your hands and knees, making sure your hands are directly under your shoulders and your knees are directly beneath your hips. Contract your abdominal muscles and keep your head in line with your spine.

2. Stretch your right arm out at shoulder height, palm facing down, as you extend your left leg out at hip height. Focus on staying as long and relaxed as possible for a slow count of ten.

3. For a more advanced move, lift your bottom foot off of the floor so it's only your knee and hand touching the floor.

4. Repeat on the opposite leg and arm.

   VARIATION: For more challenge, do this exercise balancing on your hands and knees on a step.

Push-Ups
with Feet on Step

Works: Abdominals, shoulders, and chest

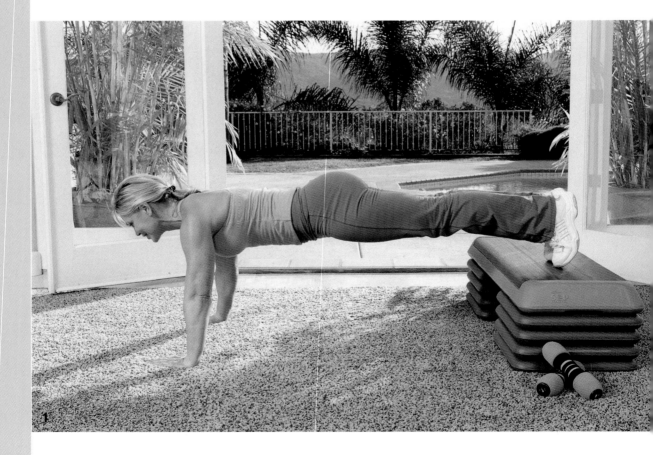

1. Place both feet on a step with both hands on the floor out from the step, hands slightly wider than your shoulders. Extend your body and arms long and straight and pull in your abdominal muscles.

2. Slowly lower your torso down toward the floor then push back up to the starting position. It's important to keep your abdominals pulled in and your head in line with your spine.

VARIATION: If it's too difficult with straight legs, bend both knees on the step.

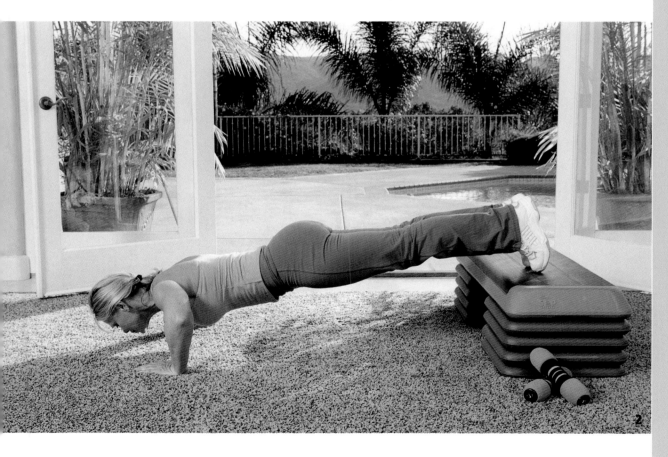

2

Side-Lying One-Arm Shoulder Lift

Works: Shoulders

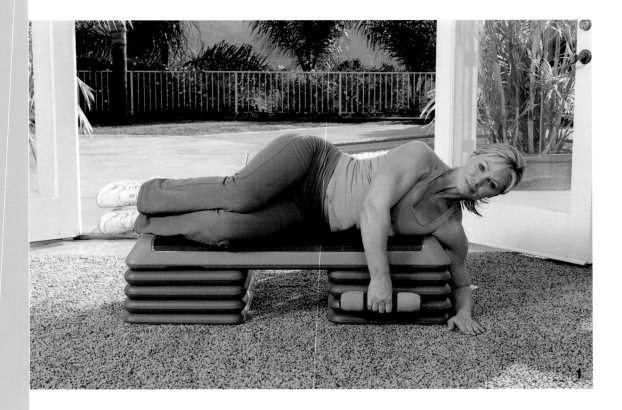

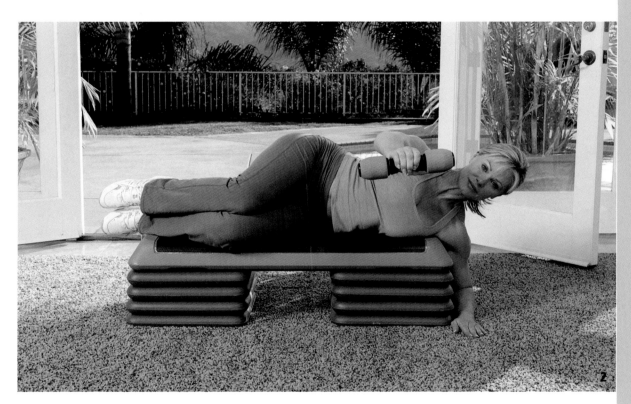

1. Lie on your left side on a step with your knees and hips bent. Hold a weight in your right hand hanging off the step in front of your torso. Rest your left forearm on the floor at the end of the step under your shoulder.

2. Slowly lift your right arm straight up to shoulder level.

3. Slowly lower and repeat for one set of reps. Repeat on the other arm.

4. Remember to keep your abdominal muscles contracted.

Plank

1. Start on the floor on your hands and knees. Place your forearms on the floor directly under your shoulders, hands together.

2. Extend your legs straight out behind you on your toes. Your body should be in a long line from your head to your toes. Keep your head in line with your spine. Make sure your hips don't sag toward the floor or stick up toward the ceiling.

3. Hold this position for thirty seconds. Remember to keep your abdominal muscles contracted, shoulders pulled back, and tailbone up.

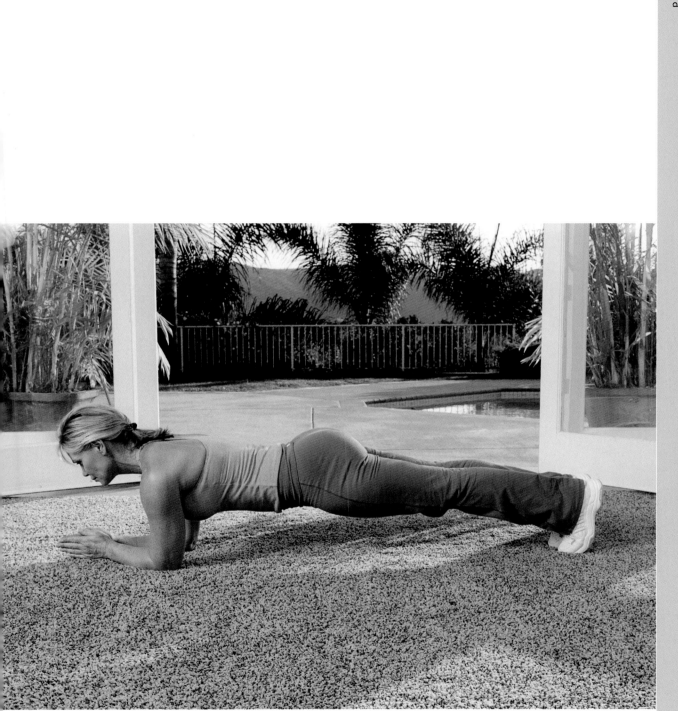

Abdominal Arcs

Works: Core, abdominals

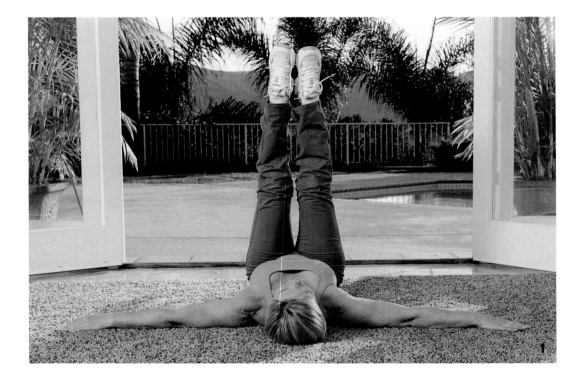

1. Lie face up on the floor with your arms stretched out to your sides at 90 degrees to your body, palms down, and your legs straight above your hips.

2. Lower your legs to one side as you look to the opposite side.

3. Return to the starting position and repeat to the other side.

   VARIATION: If straight legs are too difficult, keep your knees bent as you lower them to each side.

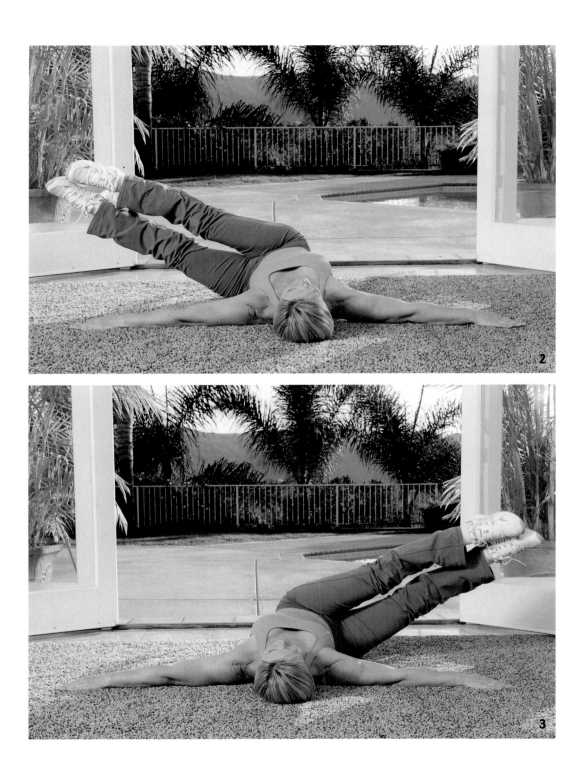

Side-Lying Obliques

Works: Abdominals, core, and obliques (sides of torso)

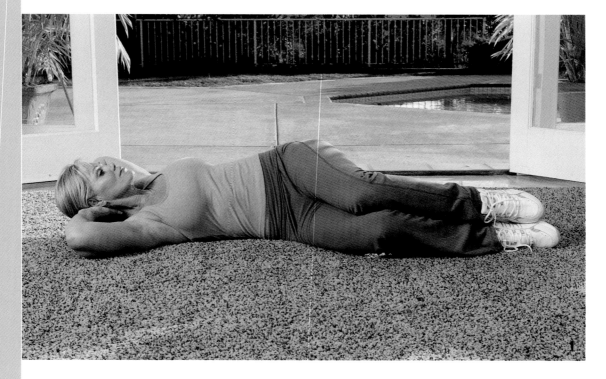

1. Lie on your back with your knees bent, both hands behind your head. Keep your torso facing up as your lower your knees to the floor on one side.

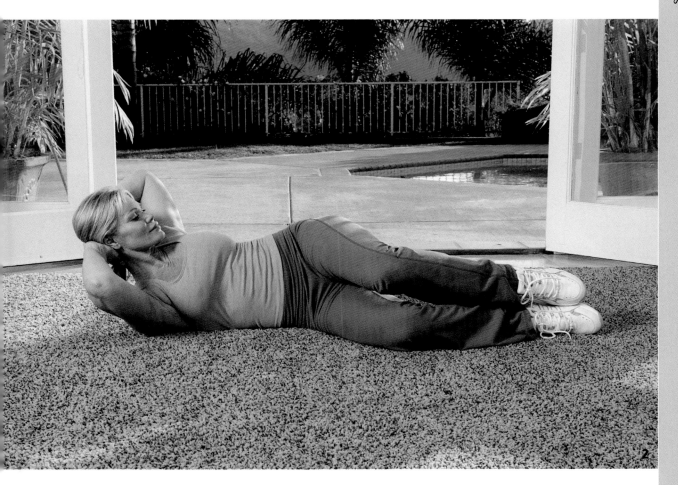

2. Lift your torso up toward the ceiling. Use your hands for support, but don't pull on your neck.

3. Return to the starting position and repeat for one set of reps. Switch sides and repeat.

Runner's Lunge

Works: Buns, thighs, and hamstrings

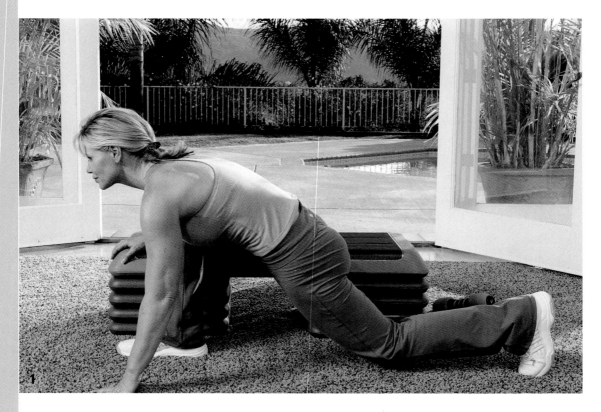

1. Kneel in a right lunge with your left leg extended back behind you. Make sure your right knee is directly over your right foot. Place your arms on each side of your right leg.

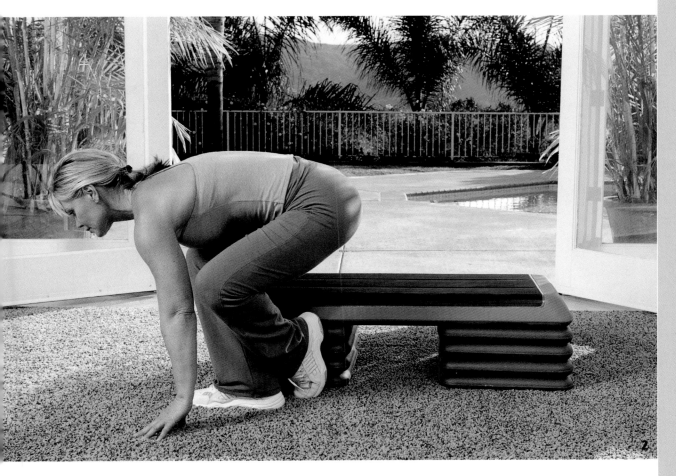

2

2. Quickly bring your left foot in behind your right foot and back out, like you are rocking forward and back off the right foot.

3. Try to keep your body down in a 90-degree angle.

4. Repeat for one set of reps then repeat on the left foot.

Dead Lifts

Works: Hamstrings, inner thighs, and lower back

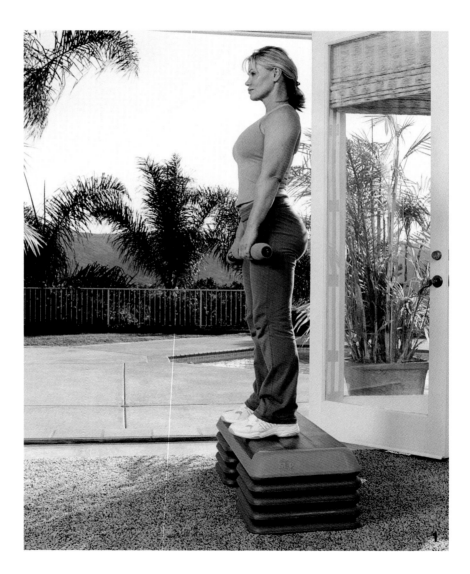

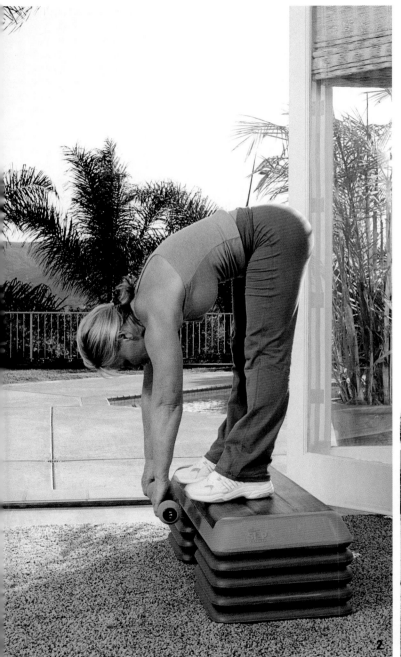

1. Stand on a step with dumbbells in both hands (this can also be done without a step), hands facing back behind you. Stand tall with your knees straight and your abdominals contracted.

2. Slowly lean forward from your hips for a count of four until your upper body is as close to the floor as your flexibility allows and your arms are hanging down in front of you. If possible, try lowering the weights past your feet.

3. Stand back up to the starting position slowly for four counts.

4. Repeat for one set of reps.

   VARIATION: If straight legs hurt your back or are too challenging, you can bend your knees slightly as you do this exercise.

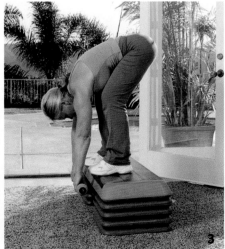

Side Leg Lifts
on Floor

Works: Outer thigh

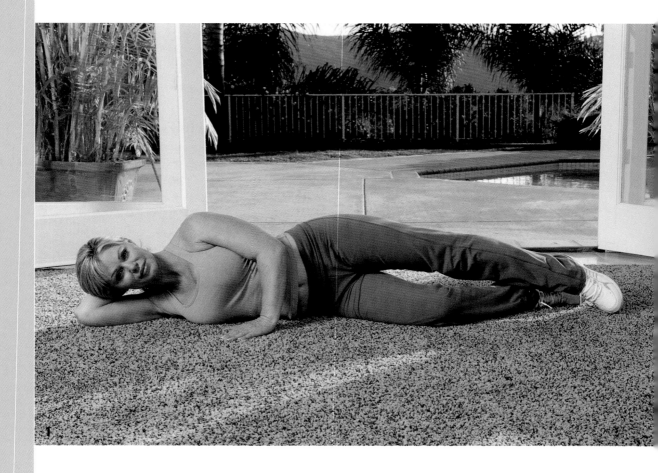

TAMILEE WEBB'S DEFY GRAVITY WORKOUT

1. Lie on your right side on the floor with your right arm under your head. Bend your right leg under your straight left leg.

2. Lift your left leg straight up toward the ceiling for two counts. Do not allow your hips to roll back; keep your left hip stacked on top of your right hip. Lower your leg back down for two counts.

3. Remember to contract your abdominal muscles.

4. Repeat for one set of reps then repeat with your right leg.

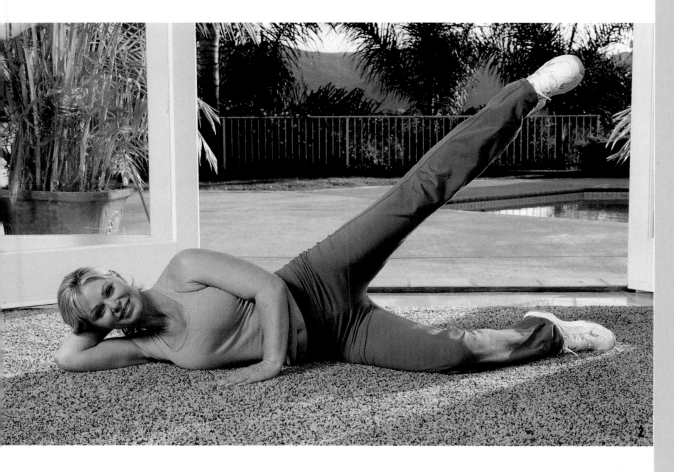

One-Legged Inner Thigh Lifts on Floor

Works: Inner thigh

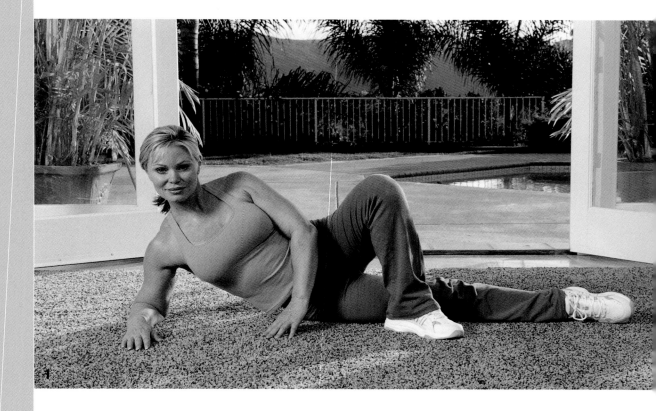

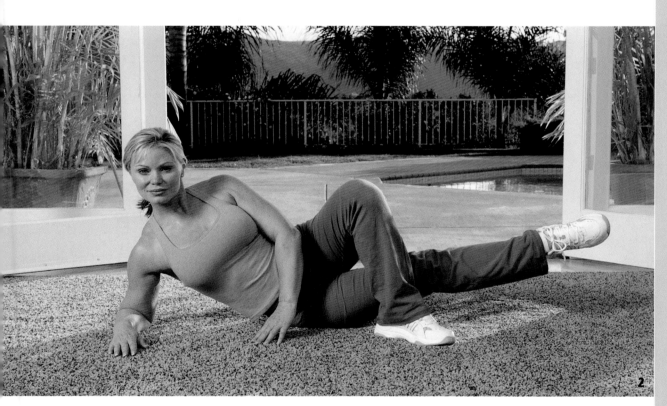

1. Lie on your right side on the floor. Cross your left leg over your extended right leg and place your left foot in front of your right knee.

2. Lift your right leg up as far as you can for two counts. Lower it back down for two counts.

3. Repeat for one set of reps then repeat with your left leg.

Prone Single Leg Lifts

Works: Buns, hamstrings, and lower back

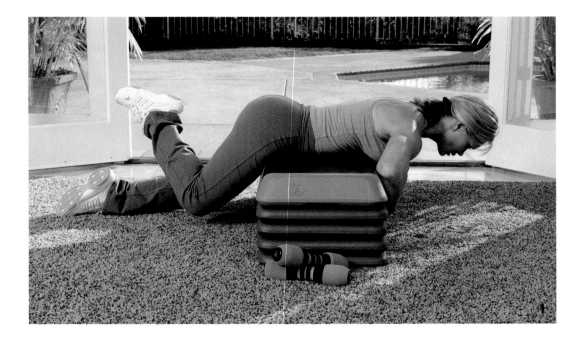

1. Lie over a step (or on the floor) with your torso on the step and your legs off the back end of it. Cross your ankles and contract your abdominal muscles.

2. Lift your right leg up off the floor to step height for two counts, then lower it back to the starting position.

3. Remember to contract your abdominal muscles and don't lift higher than is comfortable.

4. Repeat for one set of reps, alternating legs.

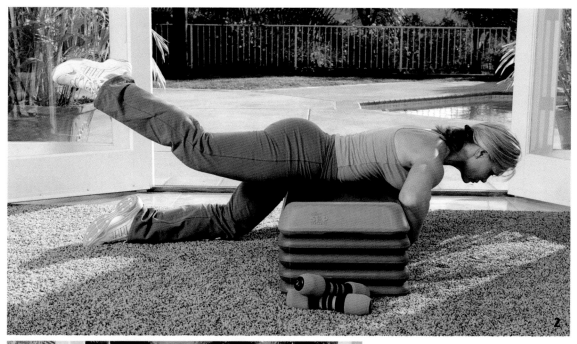

VARIATION: If you're feeling very strong, lift both legs together.

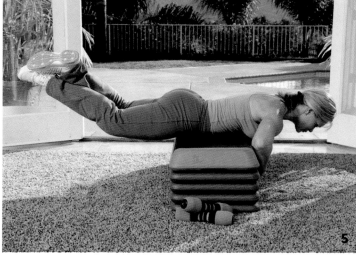

Marquee
Shoulder Lift

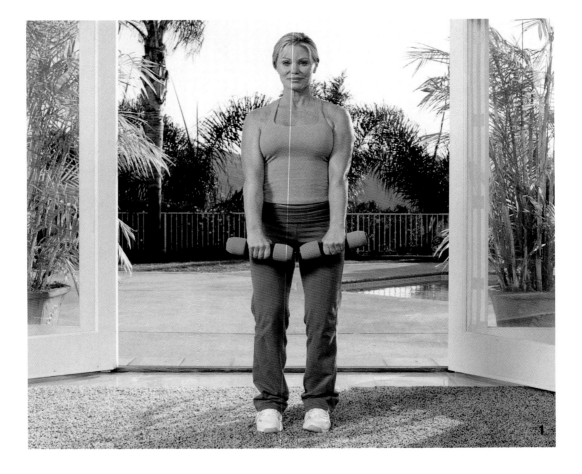

1. Stand with dumbbells in both hands by your side. Lift your arms out laterally to the side to shoulder height. Rotate and raise them overhead.

2. Slowly lower your arms back down, rotating your hands again as you pass your shoulders.

3. Keep your abdominal muscles contracted. Repeat.

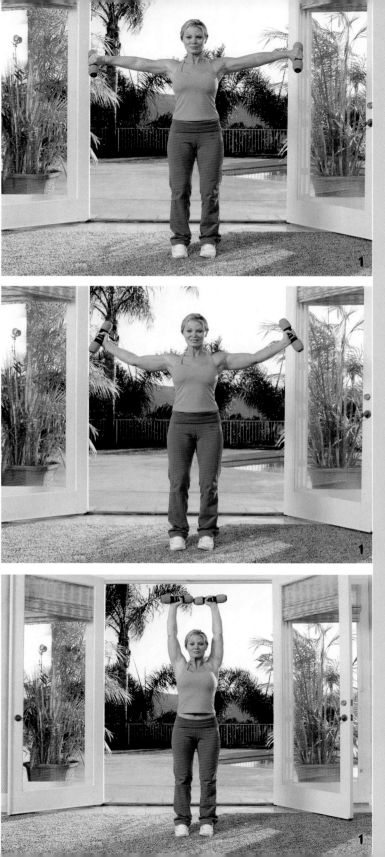

"W" Bicep Curl

Works: Biceps and front of shoulders

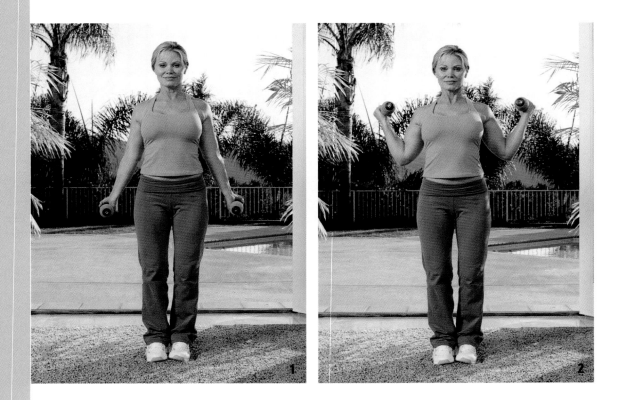

1. Stand with dumbbells in both hands by your sides, palms facing outward. Rotate your shoulders back to open up your chest.

2. Curl both arms up toward your shoulders for two counts, then down. The movement is wide and should resemble a "W." Repeat.

Rear Shoulder Raises

Works: Shoulders and triceps

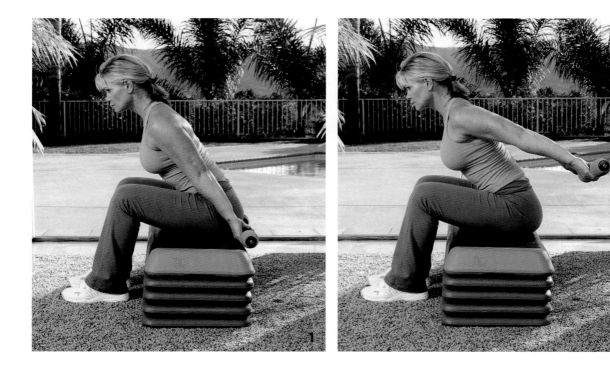

1. Sit on a step or stand with dumbbells in both hands by your side, palms facing backwards.

2. Lift both arms together behind you for two counts, then return to the starting position.

3. Keep your shoulders down and back and your abdominals contracted.

4. Repeat for one set of reps.

Overhead Tricep Extension with Elbow Squeeze

Works: Triceps and chest

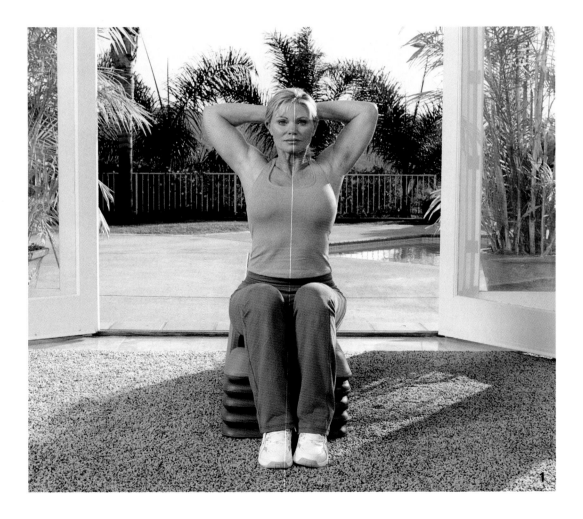

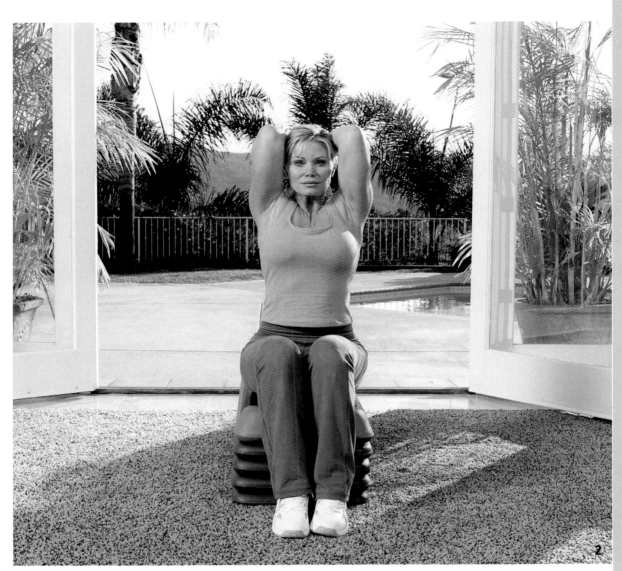

1. Sit on a step or stand with your feet together, knees bent, dumbbells in each hand behind your head, and elbows out to your side.

2. Inhale, then exhale as you slowly press your elbows toward your head. Keep your abdominal muscles pulled in.

3. Slowly return to the starting position. Repeat.

Pass The Ball Abdominal Crunch

Works: Abdominals and some chest

1. Lie on the floor and hold an exercise ball extended over your head, with your knees bent and feet on the floor. Lift your torso and the ball toward your knees as you lift your knees up off the floor toward your arms.

2. Pass the ball to your knees by placing it between your knees and squeezing it to hold it in place.

3. Extend your arms back over your head as you lower your feet back down to the floor with the ball between your legs.

4. Lift your torso and knees holding the ball back up together and pass the ball to your hands.

5. Lower back down to the starting position. Repeat for one set of reps.

   VARIATION: If you don't have a ball, grab a pillow and pass it.

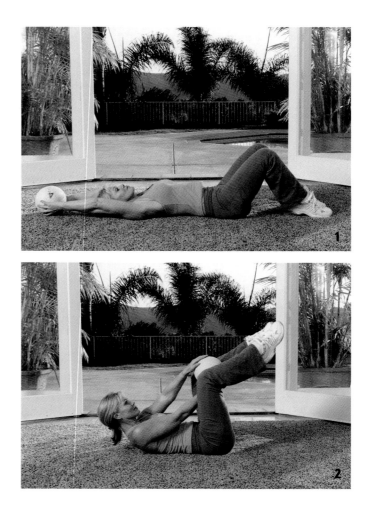

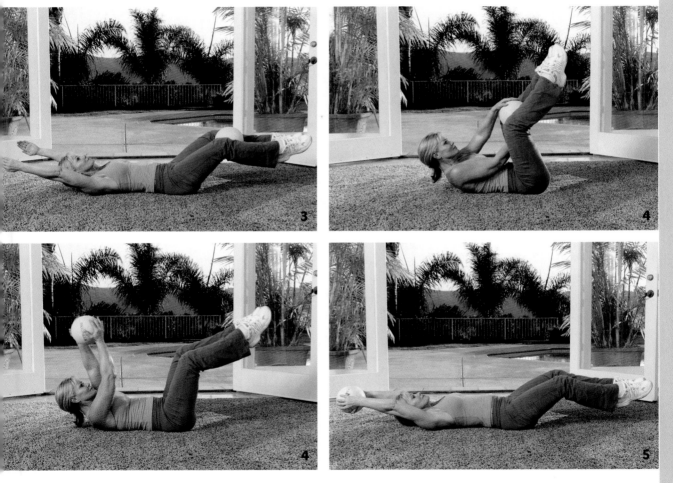

Diagonal Arm and Leg Lift

Works: Abdominals, inner thigh, and front shoulder

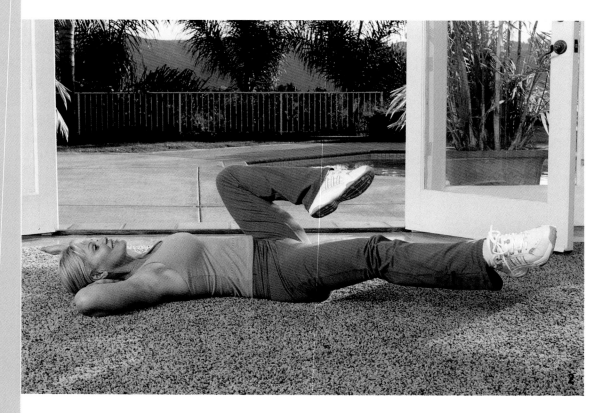

1. Lie on your back with your left knee bent. Extend your right leg out straight from your hip.

2. Put your right hand behind your head for support and extend your left arm straight out from your shoulder.

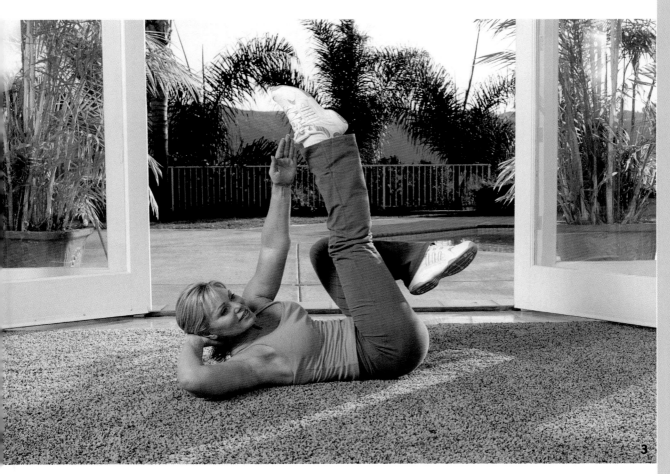

3. Lift your right leg and left arm up toward each other to meet above you. Return to the starting position.

4. Repeat for one set of reps then switch to the opposite side.

Chest Press on Step

Works: Chest and shoulders

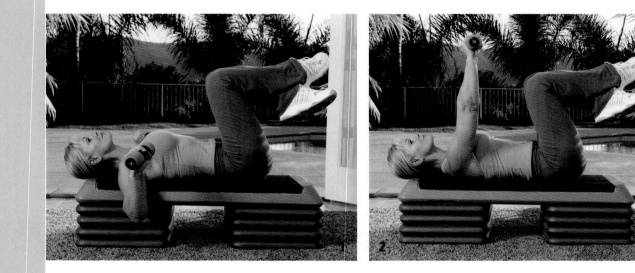

1. Lie on an exercise step or bench (or the floor) with your knees bent and hips flexed. Bend your arms and hold a dumbbell in each hand at shoulder level.

2. Press your arms straight up from your shoulders for a count of two. Bring your hands back down for a count of two.

3. Remember to keep your abdominal muscles contracted and your head in line with your spine.

4. Repeat for one set of reps.

Chest Flies on Step

Works: Chest and shoulders

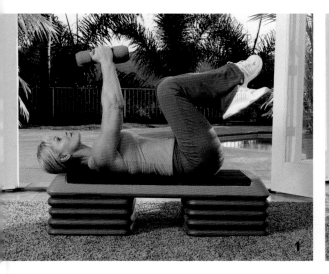 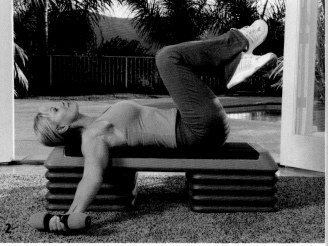

1. Lie on an exercise step or bench (or the floor) with your knees bent and hips flexed, dumbbells in each hand extended straight up from your shoulders. Slowly lower your arms out to the side with slightly flexed elbows.

2. Lower your elbows just past your shoulders then press your arms back up to the starting position.

3. Keep your head in line with your spine and your abdominal muscles contracted.

4. Repeat for one set of reps.

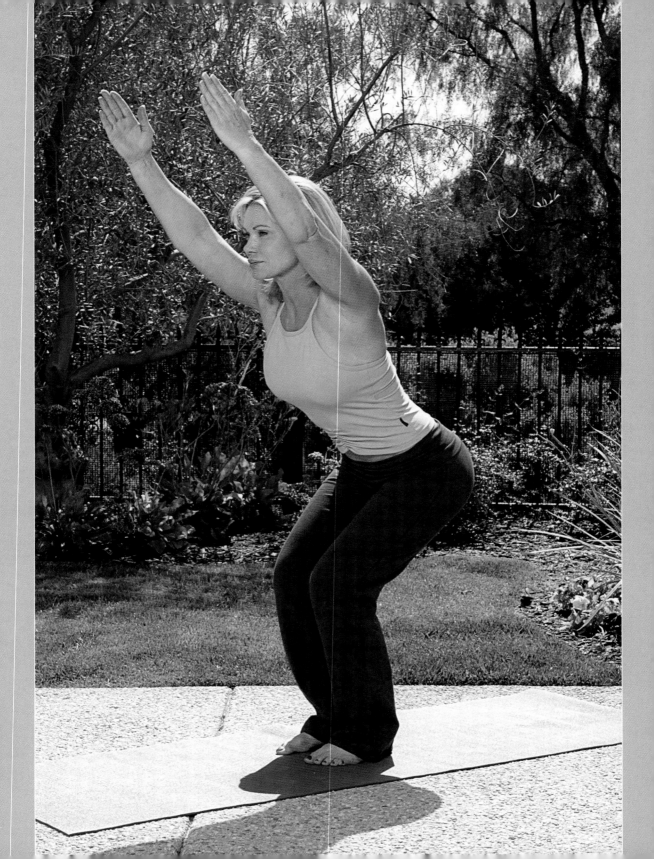

CHAPTER SIX

Yoga and Pilates Exercises

Pilates and yoga have been the hottest fitness trends in the last couple of years—and for good reason. Pilates and yoga are both considered mind/body exercises—that is, they connect your mind and spirit to the moves your body is making so that the exercise session will not only leave you fitter, but also have you feeling more relaxed and centered at the end. Of course, the other reason Pilates and yoga have been so successful is because they are so effective—Pilates creates a strong, flat torso and a longer body all around, while yoga creates strong sculpted muscles that look lean and elegant. I've been doing these exercises for years and they are a wonderful complement to the rest of the workout.

Sun Salutation

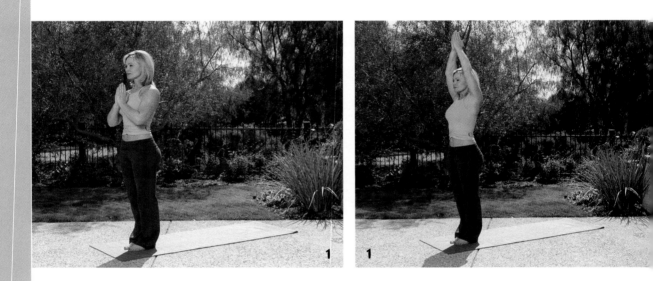

1. Begin in Mountain pose, standing straight and tall with your weight evenly distributed on both feet, with your hands in Prayer position (hands together in front of your chest, palms together, fingers pointing up). Inhale your hands up over your head, then exhale while bending forward with a flat back. Place your palms flat on the floor outside your feet (bend your knees if necessary). Tuck your chin under.

2. Inhaling, lock your elbows to support your body and jump both feet back confidently. Exhaling, straighten your legs and elbows while tightening your abdominal muscles.

3. Lower to floor, keeping torso straight, then come into an arched position with your chest on the floor your elbows lifted.

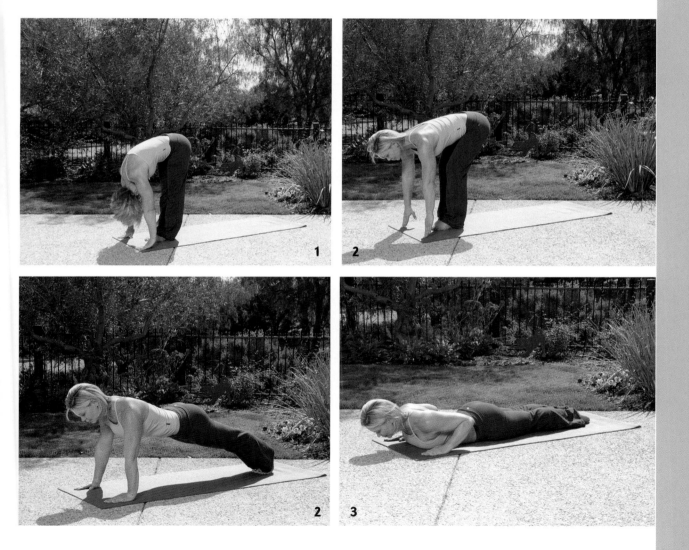

Sun Salutation (cont.)

4. Inhaling, slide your body forward and up. Exhaling, drop your hips to the floor, press your arms straight, stretch up through your head, and arch your back. Keep your legs together and press the tops of your feet into the floor. Imagine that you are trying to push your hips through your elbows to increase the arch in your back. Hold this pose for two breaths.

5. Inhaling, tuck your toes under and bring your feet close together. Exhaling, push up onto your feet and hands, drop your head between your shoulders, lift your hips to the ceiling to create an inverted "V" shape (this is the well-known Downward Dog position), and press your heels toward the floor to stretch your hamstrings. Extend as long as you can all the way up through your spine and down through your heels.

6. Inhaling, step your right foot forward between your hands into a lunge. If you cannot hold the lunge position, drop your left knee to the floor. Look forward, and lengthen through your chest.

7. Exhaling and maintaining your leg position, straighten your back. Rest both hands on your left thigh, one on top of the other.

8. Inhaling, circle your arms overhead, and bring your palms together. Interlock your fingers, with your index fingers pointing up. Exhaling, arch your back and sink deeply into the lunge.

9. Inhaling, bend forward and place your palms flat on the floor on either side of your foot. Exhaling, step your left foot forward to meet your right foot. Drop your upper body down to your thighs, with your chin tucked under. Straighten both legs.

10. Inhaling, come up with a straight back and lift your arms to the side to shoulder height. Exhaling, bring your hands together in front of your chest, palms together, fingers pointing up. Close your eyes. Inhale deeply and slowly, and release your hands to your sides.

11. Complete the sequence six times, alternating legs in the lunge.

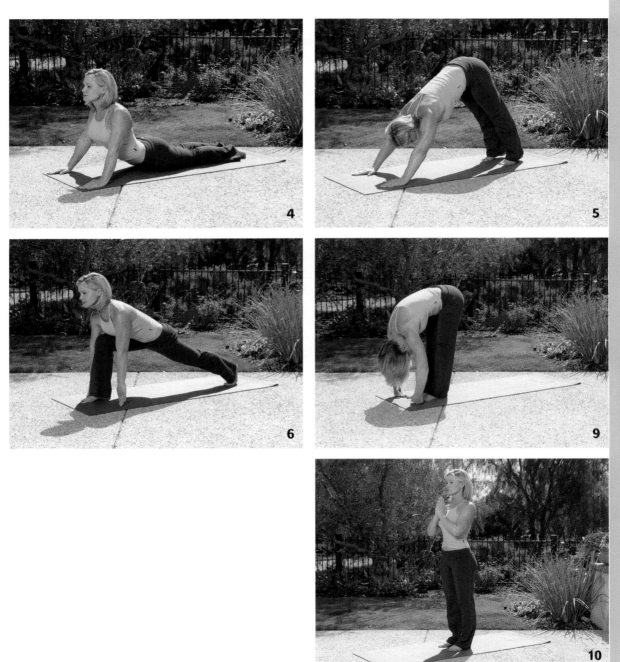

Chair Pose

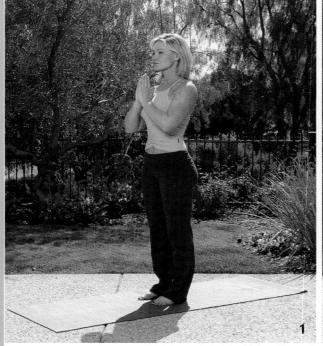
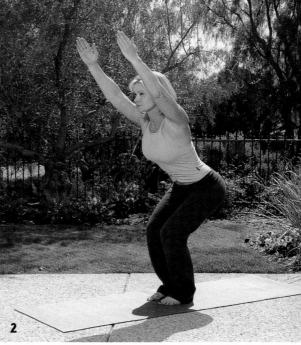

1. Stand with your feet together and hands in Prayer position. Lean slightly forward at the hips and raise your arms overhead.

2. Bend your knees a few inches and press your legs together as you lengthen your arms upward as far as you comfortably can. Breathe deeply as you hold for several breaths.

Toes in the Water

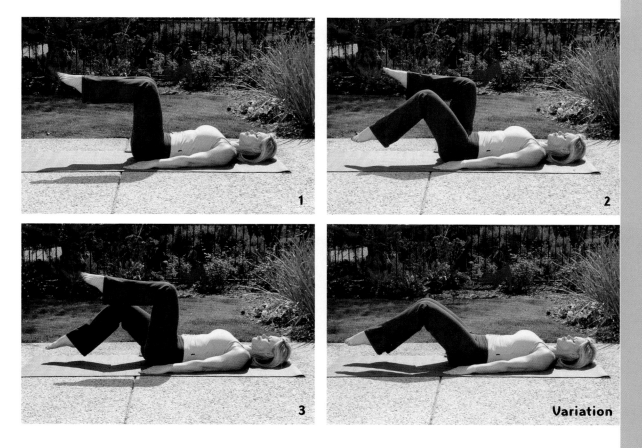

1. Lie on your back, legs bent in the air with your knees above your hips.

2. Lower your left foot down toward the floor without moving your hips or torso (as if you're dipping a toe in the water).

3. Repeat, alternating legs.

   VARIATION: For an added challenge, try dipping both toes in the water.

135

Dead Bug

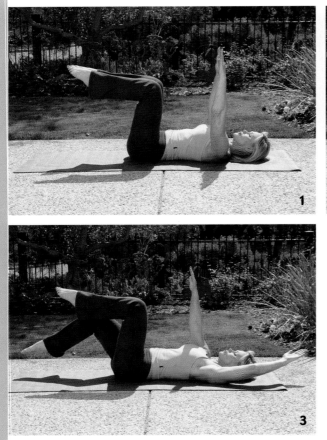

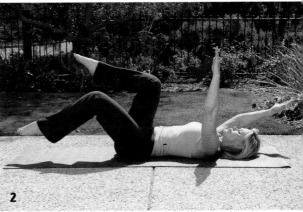

1. Lie on your back, knees above your hips and arms extended up, hands directly over your shoulders.

2. Lower your right arm and left toe toward the ground in opposite directions.

3. Repeat, alternating opposite arms and legs.

Side Plank

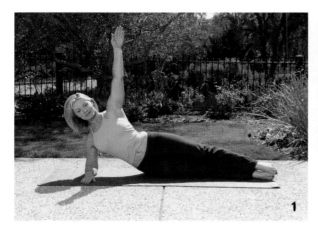

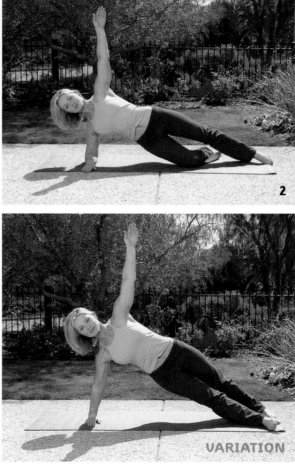

1. Lie on your right side, leaning on your right forearm.

2. Bend your bottom leg and come up into a plank by lifting your body off the floor, keeping your torso straight. Extend your left arm up from your shoulder.

3. Move your shoulders away from your ears, lengthening your spine.

   VARIATION: You can also do this with both legs straight and your bottom arm straight.

4. Repeat on the left side.

Reed

1. Begin in Mountain pose with your hands in Prayer position. Reach your arms over your head.

2. Inhale, pull your shoulders down, tuck your pelvis under, and contract your abdominal muscles as you bend from the waist toward your right. The goal is to remain in the same plane as your legs and hips; don't twist or bend your torso to the front or back.

3. Hold this pose for a few breaths, then straighten up on an exhalation. Take a breath while stancing upright and then bend to the left without tilting forward or back.

4. Inhale and check that your shoulders are lowered and your abdominal muscles are contracted, then tuck your pelvis under as you tilt backwards, leading with the crown of your head and not bending at your neck or waist. Strive to keep the line of your body long and elegant. Hold this pose for a few breaths, and on an inhalation, return to standing straight.

5. Exhale, reach up and then forward, coming into a forward bend, bending from your hips and reaching your hands to the floor alongside your feet.

6. Inhale and return to standing with your arms above your head. Exhale and bring your arms down.

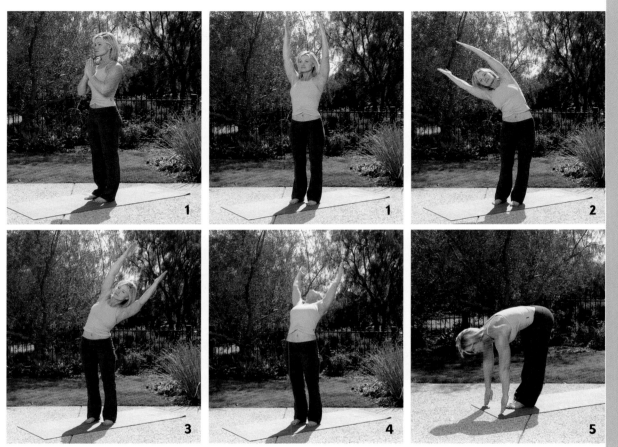

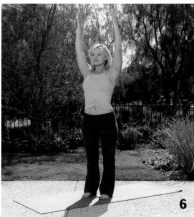

Bridge

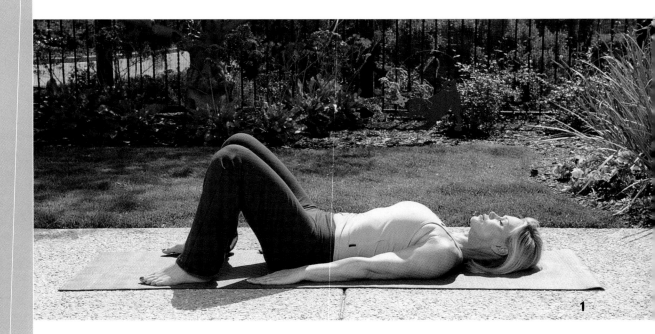

1

1. Lie on the floor with your knees bent and your feet flat on the floor, heels as close to your bottom as comfortably possible.

2. Exhale and press your inner feet and arms actively into the floor as you lift your hips upwards. Keep your thighs and inner feet parallel to one another.

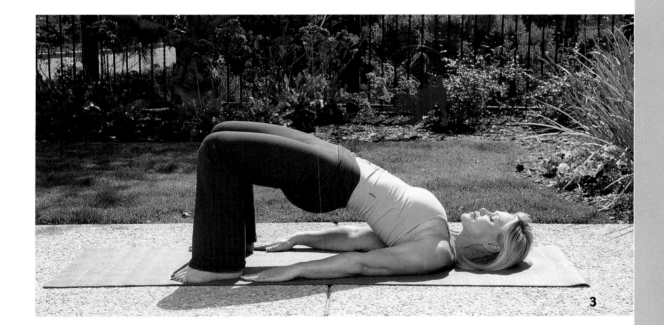

3.

3. Lift your hips until your thighs are about parallel to the floor. Keep your knees directly over your heels. Lengthen your tailbone toward the backs of your knees.

4. Lift your chin slightly away from your sternum and, firming your shoulder blades against your back, press the top of your sternum toward your chin. Firm your outer arms, broaden your shoulder blades, and try to lift the space between them at the base of your neck up into your torso.

5. Release with an exhalation, rolling your spine slowly down onto the floor. Never turn your head in this pose.

Locust

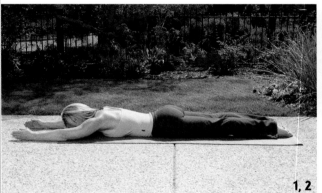 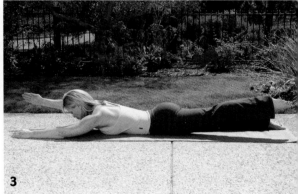

1, 2   3

1. Lie face down on the floor with your arms above your head, palms facing each other and forehead down.

2. Bring your knees and ankles together. Squeeze your shoulder blades together and down. Push your pinkie fingers into the floor. Pull your abdominal muscles inward, contract your butt muscles, and press your hips firmly into the floor.

3. On your next inhalation, raise your head, right arm, and left leg to a comfortable height. Extend out through your head, fingers, and toes.

4. As you breathe, allow your limbs to move with your breath. In other words, don't hold your breath or try to hold your limbs still. Instead, focus on breathing deeply.

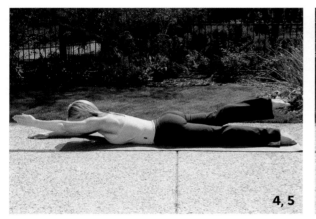
4, 5

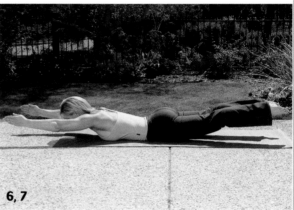
6, 7

5. Exhale as you slowly lower your arm and leg. Take another full breath and on your next inhalation, raise your left arm and right leg. Exhale and lower them slowly.

6. Lower your face to the floor. Take another full breath and raise both legs away from the floor, keeping your face lowered. Once again, let your breath lead your body.

7. Extend the front of your body as you pull your shoulder blades together, raising your head, arms, and upper torso away from the floor. Look straight ahead, opening the front of your chest.

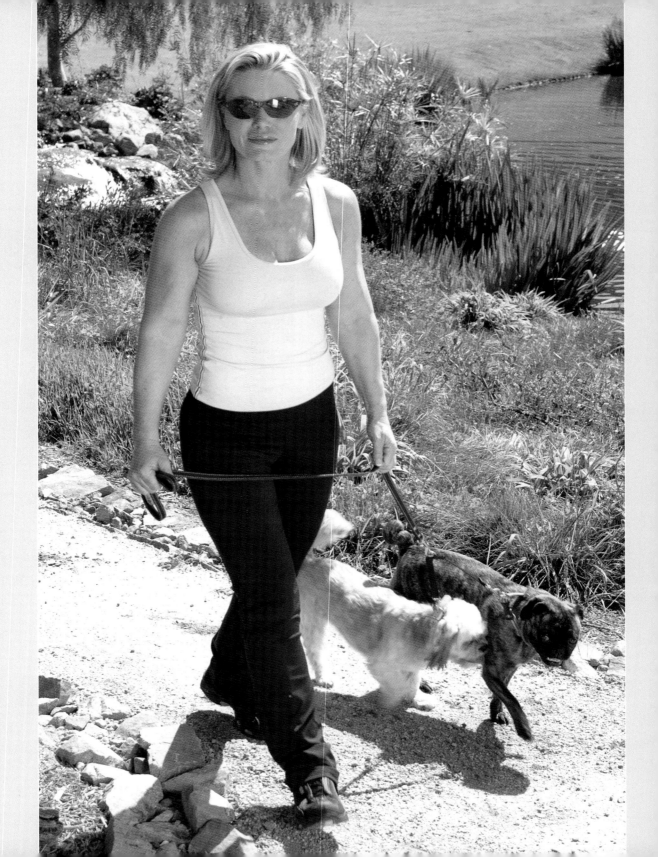

CHAPTER SEVEN

Nutritional Goals for Each Week

Too many women believe they have to cut foods out of their diet in order to lose weight, but really, the best way to change your eating habits (and thus lose weight) is to adopt healthy eating habits which will naturally replace the unhealthy eating you've been doing.

By the end of the program, these habits will be second nature. Of course, not every day of your life will be filled with perfect eating, but once you know these eight basic rules of healthy eating, you'll be able to plan your meals more effectively.

Healthy Eating Habit—Week Three

Write down what you eat.

Keeping track of exactly what you eat every day is one of the top ten tricks of people who lose weight and keep it off for a long time, according to researchers. There are a lot of reasons for this. First, if you write down what you eat, you won't consume a lot of calories unconsciously. Second, you'll actually be able to see where your diet is going off track (you may think it's the eggs you're having for breakfast, but then, once you've written everything down, you'll see that you're consuming 300 calories in chocolate during work). Finally, writing down what you eat will help you make better choices even before you put the food in your mouth (we'll talk more about this next week).

You can buy a food journal at most book stores (look in the nutrition section), but you should also feel free to simply write down what you eat on any piece of paper (or enter it into your computer). The most important thing you'll need, besides honesty (and that's really important) is some information on calorie counts and other nutritional information, such as fat and carbs. To find these, you can get a book such as any of Corinne Netzer's *Calorie Counters,* or you can go online and simply input the food you've eaten. Or, you can go online to a website such as **www.calorie-count.com.**

You will have to be honest not only about what you eat, but also about how much you eat of each and every food. Even if it's "just one Hershey kiss" or "just a handful of peanuts," write it down and add the calories into your daily total. For some people, unconscious eating keeps their weight higher than they would like. A handful of a snack and a couple of Hershey kisses every day can add up to hundreds of unwanted calories, which can, in turn, end up as extra pounds on your body.

Another thing that some people like to keep track of in a food journal is how they feel when they eat. Some of us are emotional eaters. That is, we eat not for nutrition or to satisfy hunger, but to soothe a feeling, such as sadness or fear. If you suspect that emotional eating is a problem for you, write down how you feel at each meal (or between meals) as a part of your food journal.

In the end, these are the elements you will need in your journal:

* Food
* Quantity
* Time eaten (or for which meal)
* Calorie
* Fat
* Fiber
* Protein
* Carbohydrate
* **Total**

Your Journal should look something like this:

	CALORIES	CARBS	PROTEIN	FAT	FIBER
Breakfast					
2 scrambled eggs	202	2.6	13.6	14.8	–
1 Tbsp butter	67	0	0.1	7.6	–
Whole wheat toast	78	14.6	3.1	1.4	2.1
8 oz. orange juice	112	25.6	1.6	0.8	–
¼ cup 2% Milk	30.5	2.9	2	1.2	–
Snack					
2 handfuls M&Ms	103	15.5	1	4.4	0.5
Snack					
Carrot sticks	65	13.8	1.4	0.9	3.1
Lunch					
Tuna melt	301	4	12	13	–
Salad with	33	6.7	2.6	0.1	–
2 Tbsp reduced-fat dressing	22	0.7	0.1	1	–
Dinner					
Chef's salad	620	8	64	37	–
Snack					
1 cup coffee chip ice cream	340	34	6	20	–
TOTAL	**1,672.50**	**128.4**	**107.8**	**104**	**6.5**

As you can see, our sample woman has learned that she is taking in way too much fat and far too little fiber. Her calorie count is pretty good, though, so she just needs to make some changes such as having a high-fiber snack instead of M&Ms, and making sure she has high-fiber vegetables in her salad, rather than fatty meats and cheeses.

Other things you might want to write down: how much you've exercised, how you feel when you eat, if you've had enough water, and anything that pertains to your particular diet goals (such as getting enough fiber, calcium, or your carb counts).

Healthy Eating Habit—Week Four

Plan what you eat.

Now that you've taken a look at what you've been eating, it's time to get to the next step: planning as many healthy meals and snacks as you can. I firmly believe that no one can reach a goal until they have a plan to get them there. You have to know how you're going to get from here to there. So, before the day begins (at least, that's what works for me—I make up my eating plan the night before) figure out what you're going to eat for breakfast, lunch, dinner, and for your snacks. And then, figure out how you're going to make that plan into reality.

For example, if you decide you're going to have a salad for lunch, are you going to make it in the morning and bring it to the office? Or are you going to go out? Leaving your food choices to make until the last minute is a recipe for disaster (sorry for the pun) because it leaves you vulnerable to eating whatever is available, and often those choices aren't nutritious, or even satisfying.

Be specific and, also, try to count the calories and other nutritional information for the foods you plan to eat. You might find that you really aren't eating enough during the day, which is why you're so hungry at night. Or, maybe you'll see that there is actually plenty of room in your eating plan for a piece of candy in the late afternoon.

Now, it won't always be possible to stick with your eating plan, but the good news is that if you have a plan, you will be more likely to be conscious of what you eat so that when unexpected things happen your diet won't be thrown completely off track.

Healthy Eating Habit—Week Five

Add fruits and vegetables.

Now that you've become more conscious of what you're eating and, hopefully, weaned yourself of some processed foods, it's time to make sure you're eating the right amount of fruits and vegetables.

According to the Department of Agriculture, which created the Food Pyramid many of us know, we should eat five to nine servings of fruits and vegetables each day. But, I have to say, there is no way to eat too many of these foods, and I try to center each of my meals and snacks around a fruit or vegetable. For example, when I'm planning breakfast, I make sure that my cereal has fruit in it or that my scrambled eggs have peppers and onions. My snacks range from raisins to cherry tomatoes with cheese or celery with peanut butter.

Most people snack on snack food, such as chips or pretzels, but those foods have no nutritional value. But, if you are conscious about making sure you're eating enough fruits and vegetables, then you'll find you won't need to eat those unhealthy foods and your weight will be under control.

Also, fruits and vegetables are very low in calories and high in nutrients, so you can eat a lot of them without gaining weight. People who stay away from "high-sugar" vegetables or fruits, such as carrots and bananas, don't understand that no one has ever gotten fat from eating too many of these foods. It's almost impossible to overeat fruits and vegetables because they are so satisfying.

Healthy Eating Habit—Week Six

Add protein.

We used to center our meals around carbohydrates (such as pasta or rice), but these days, with the acceptance of low-carb diets, we realize that the proper amount of protein will help us keep our weight in check, as well as keep us satisfied. And, meanwhile, protein will help our muscles stay strong, so that all of our weight training will pay off and we'll have great new shapes.

Protein should be a part of every meal and snack (just like fruits and vegetables). You won't need a lot of protein-rich foods to feel full—two or three cheese cubes, two slices of turkey, a hard-boiled egg. They all have high amounts of protein without being too high in calories.

You have to be careful about two things when you're working protein into your eating plan: portion size and fat. If you're having steak for dinner, you need to make sure it's a proper-sized piece (three ounces) rather than the oversized options so many restaurants (and homes) offer these days. Meat, chicken, cheese, and other high protein foods are high in both calories and fat (especially the saturated kind which isn't good for our hearts) and so they must be eaten in moderation. Even the Atkins people acknowledge this now.

Healthy Eating Habit—Week Seven

Eat calcium.

Calcium is a mineral that makes up your bones and keeps them strong. Ninety-nine percent of the calcium in your body is stored in your bones and teeth. The remaining one percent is in your blood and soft tissues—without it, your muscles wouldn't contract correctly, your blood wouldn't clot, and your nerves wouldn't carry messages. It is mainly the calcium in your diet that protects the calcium in your bones. Your body actually tears down and builds bone all of the time in order to make its calcium available for your body's functions. If you don't get enough calcium from the food you eat, your body automatically takes the calcium you need from your bones. If your body continues to tear down more bone than it replaces over a period of years, your bones become weak and break easily. This leads to osteoporosis, which affects approximately twenty-five million American women.

The most available source of calcium in our food supply comes from milk and foods made with milk. The Food Pyramid recommends 2-3 servings from the milk, yogurt, and cheese food group every day. Women need to get 1,000 milligrams of calcium a day and 1,200 milligrams after the age of fifty-one. Most Americans do not eat the recommended number of servings of calcium-rich foods to get the calcium they need.

Calcium is also found in foods such as dark green vegetables, nuts, grains, beans, canned salmon, and sardines (if you eat the bones). These foods can help contribute to your calcium quota. But without dairy in your diet, it may be difficult to meet your daily calcium requirements.

Non-fat or low-fat dairy products provide the easiest, most plentiful sources of calcium. In addition, try adding broccoli, kale, and salmon, especially with the bones included, to your diet. Many processed foods are now fortified with calcium, including fruit juices, snack foods, and breakfast cereals. You might find the easiest way to get the daily calcium you need is to make changes in your diet and take a calcium supplement.

The key is to choose a supplement that you will actually take every day. Taking a supplement at mealtime is a convenient way to remember your daily calcium. The most common type of supplement, calcium carbonate such as Os-Cal, is even more effective if taken with a meal. Calcium carbonate is inexpensive and provides moreelemental calcium (what the body actually uses) than other supplements, such as calcium citrate and calcium lactate. Certain calcium antacids, such as Tums, are a good, inexpensive source of calcium. The National Osteoporosis Foundation has recommended Tums as an excellent source of calcium.

Calcium will also help you keep your weight at the right level. As dietary calcium intake increases, it acts at the cellular level to alter energy metabolism so that more food energy is burned and less is stored as fat, according to researchers at the University of Tennessee's Department of Nutrition. Their third National Health and Nutrition Examination Survey (NHANES III) shows an inverse relationship between calcium and dairy intakes and body fat in adults. The researchers concluded that low calcium diets lead to increased fat storage and higher calcium diets favor increased burning of fat.

Healthy Eating Habit—Week Eight

Plan your fabulous treats.

I would never give up chocolate. I firmly believe that women (or, at least, most women) need chocolate, just as Debra Waterhouse has written. But, also, as she advises, I believe in self-indulgence, not over-indulgence. The problem most people have with chocolate (or any of their favorite foods, especially those that aren't that nutritious) is that they try to stop eating it altogether rather than finding a healthy way to incorporate it into their eating plans.

In other words, I believe that, in the same way you're going to pay attention to how much you eat, as well as the details of what you eat (protein, fruits and vegetables, and fat), I also think you need to pay attention to—and enjoy—the foods you love simply because they taste good.

Here are some of my tricks. I keep chocolates in my house, but I only eat them when I really want them. Because I know that I can have them whenever I want, they don't have a hold over me and I rarely eat too many (more than two or three Hershey's Kisses, for example). If I go out to dinner with my girlfriends—one of my favorite things to do—we all share a great piece of cake for dessert. But, I don't do this every night, because I know that I will be able to have my cake when I really want it.

If you have a favorite treat, such as ice cream, you need to figure out how you're going to incorporate it into your eating plan in such a way that it won't cause you to gain weight—and that *is* possible. If you eat three to five well-planned meals throughout the day, you'll have plenty of room for the extra calories of a small slice of cake, some chocolate, or a dish of ice cream.

Just remember to think about portion size and the calorie count, as well as fat and carbs if you're counting them, too.

You may need to take other non-nutritious foods out of your diet to fit your favorite into your eating plan. For example, if you regularly have a bagel for breakfast but also want to eat chocolate ice cream after dinner, you might need to change your bagel to whole-wheat toast in the morning. This way, your calorie count won't be too high and you'll still be able to have your favorite treat.

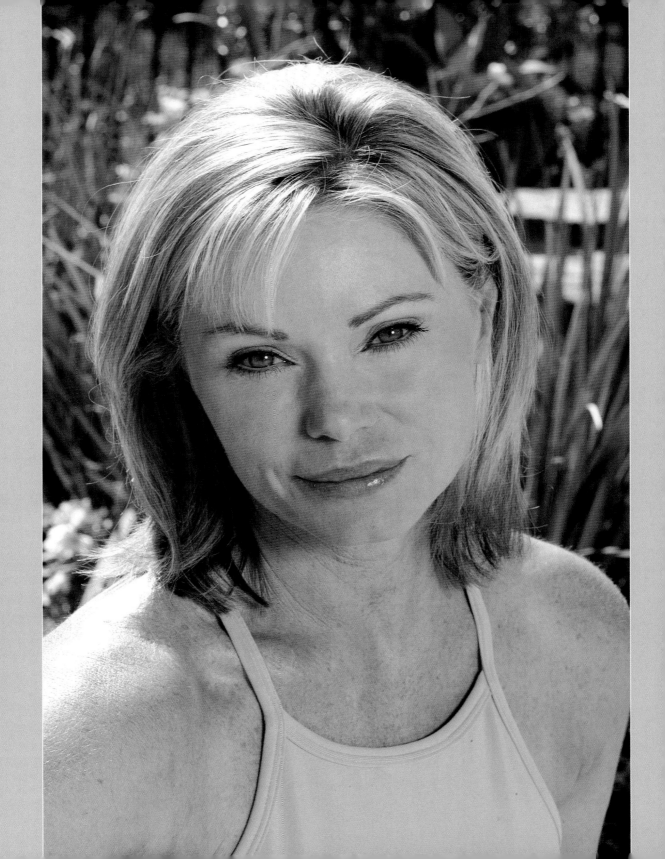

CHAPTER EIGHT

Taking Care of Your Outside

Skin Care and Beauty Treatments

"Who Are You?"

That's not something you would ever think you would ask, but there you are... posing this question as you stare back at this face in the foggy bathroom mirror after your morning shower. Where did your sharp jaw line go? Where did these forehead wrinkles come from? You didn't have these freckles and age spots a few years ago!

Gravity and aging not only affect your muscles and bones, but also your skin. All of a sudden it seems that you can read the story of your life in each dark circle, wrinkle, and droop of your skin—not to mention the trails that the crows have been creating as they tread across your tired eyes. Couple those issues with dry skin, not-so pearly whites, and varicose veins, and you are a walking tribute to Father Time, though you look more like your mother or grandmother.

Skin is our largest organ, consisting of billions of cells that are constantly being regenerated. When we're born, our skin is smooth, soft and flawless, but as we age our skin changes due to nutrition, hormones, sun, and other environmental factors.

There are three layers to the skin: the top layer, or the *epidermis;* the middle layer, or the *dermis;* and the bottom layer, or *subcutaneous tissue.*

* The epidermis is the skin we see. It contains dead cells that are replaced every three to five weeks. Believe it or not, over your lifetime, you will shed about ninety pounds of dead skin!

* The dermis is the thickest of the three layers and contains nerves, blood vessels, fibers, glands, collagen, and elastin. This is where wrinkles begin (and end with proper maintenance). Collagen is responsible for the structural support, while elastin is in charge of the firmness of the skin.

* Subcutaneous tissue is the bottom layer and is made up mostly of fat. It supports and protects against trauma and regulates hot body temperature.

The Culprits

Your twenties and thirties are a great time to cleanse and moisturize, but once you get into your forties, there's more to taking care of your skin than just cleansing and moisturizing. There are new issues that you have to face, so to speak.

Over the years our skin is exposed to many environmental factors like sun exposure, smog, smoke, and other chemical toxins that can cause damage. Skin loses its ability to regenerate elasticity and collagen, which helps keep the skin firm. This is where you need to help it by building up the collagen through topical creams and treatments.

A perfect example of how environment affects your skin is smoke. A person who smokes will have dry, grayish looking skin that is more wrinkled than a person who doesn't smoke.

What we put into our body can also affect the quality of our skin. Diet plays a big role in the how our skin ages and looks. Foods rich in antioxidants help fight free radicals (which we discussed in chapter 1).

Drugs, whether prescription, over the counter, or illegal, can all have an effect on the look and overall health of our skin and body. Have you ever seen a person who has done years of hard drugs? They look much older than they really are because the body is not getting the proper care and nutrients it needs to rebuild the cells. Many anti-depression medications will cause weight gain, while still other medications can dry out your skin (yet another good reason to drink lots of water).

It is no new news to tell a teenager that hormones affect their skin. They know full well that they go hand-in-hand. And it is still true in adulthood. There isn't much that can be done about hormones when you're a teenager, but women with hormonal imbalances that are causing skin problems can seek help to find some type of solution.

And last, but certainly not least, let's not forget about stress! Stress, the almighty emotion, can affect more than just our skin (see chapter 1 for Stress Factors). This is where exercise, meditation, and healthy eating can ease the daily stress our lives and contribute to a healthy body covered in healthy skin.

Habits That Age Us

There are little things we do throughout the day that can add years to our face. These habits can be responsible for premature aging. The best way to check if you are guilty of these habits is to have a friend keep an eye out for them. If you are, then ask yourself what makes you do them.

1. *Squinting:* Leads to crow's feet and can deepen lines around the eyes. Do you need new glasses or maybe sunglasses?

2. *Rubbing eyes:* Continuous eye rubbing can break down the tissues of the eyelids and cause loose skin. Do you have allergies?

3. *Frowning:* Turning down the corners of your mouth can lead to horrible lines around your lips.

4. *Sleeping on your side:* This can actually stretch the skin on your face, leading to more wrinkles.

5. *Poor posture:* can cause double chins, potbellies, and swayback…not to mention adding years to your figure. To check for good posture, try the following test. Stand sideways in front of a mirror. Your ears, shoulders, and hips should be in line with one another. Turn to face the mirror and let your arms hang naturally. If you can see the backs of your hands, your shoulders are too rounded forward.

6. *Smoking:* The constant pursing motion of your mouth for each drag leads to those vertical lines around your lips. Smoking also slows the blood flow in your body, which can leave you looking sallow and worn out.

Here are a few tips on how to help avoid these problems:

1. Wear sunglasses. Not only does this protect the delicate skin around your eyes from the sun's harmful rays, but it helps you to avoid squinting. Try wearing a darker lens rather than the clear to lighter colors that fashion dictates as "cool" this season.

2. Sleeping face-up can reduce puffy eyes and sleep lines that make you look older than you really are. Try sleeping with your head a little higher, so that the fluid build-up in your eye area is minimal. Experiment with this for two weeks and see the difference.

My skin was still healing. Because I was a healthy patient, my healing progress was coming along nicely. Every day my skin looked better and better. By the end of the third week, my face had pink fresh new skin. Eight years later, although I'm sure the procedure is better now than when I had it done, I still would not want to go through another Co2 laser. That is why I take such good care of my skin now. I got another chance to take care of something that I didn't think too much about while I was young. But it is precisely during those younger years when you should plan ahead.

Today people comment quite frequently on my skin. Some have even suggested that I have had a face lift (which I have not). I cannot say whether I will have one in the future, but for now I have a skin care program that I follow to help keep my skin healthy looking. One of my students, Neala, a woman with beautiful skin, is my aesthetician. She oversees my facials, educates me on what's new, and recommends special treatments if she feels my skin is in need of a little extra assistance and care. I see her once a month for a facial to help clean my pores and leave my face glowing.

A very important tip that she has given me is to treat your neck, chest, and face the same when it comes to skin care. Nothing says, "I'm aging," like a crepe-y neck, so be sure to follow the moisturizing and cleansing programs for the delicate skin of your chest and neck, as well as your face.

My Skin Care Program

Morning Routine

1. Exfoliate every morning (or at least five times a week) with a citrus herbal cleanser with a fine grain. This lightly lifts dead skin so my skin will better receive the other products I put on.

2. Dry skin thoroughly. Pat; never rub.

3. Apply a collagen product (either Lucrece collagen serum or Epicuren).

4. Apply a topical Vitamin C product.

5. Apply an eye cream. Amino acid-based products are great as they tighten and firm. Be careful with the delicate tissues around your eyes. Pat on the cream with your ring finger. Never drag your finger across your skin.

6. Spritz on protein toner.

7. Apply moisturizer with sunscreen.

8. Apply makeup.

Evening Routine

1. Remove makeup.

2. Cleanse skin.

3. Spritz on protein toner.

4. Apply eye cream and moisturizer (amino acid with vitamin A is best for tightening the skin).

These days, when we are juggling schedules and it's hard to find time to wash our faces at night, there are ways around it. Do your nighttime face cleansing and moisturizing routine before dinner. Then it's done. The worst thing for your skin is to go to bed with makeup on. Whether you use a cream or a gel cleanser, wash with a washcloth. The light abrasiveness will help to remove all the dirt and makeup off your face. For some of you, it might seem like a lot, but it only takes a few minutes. A few minutes is worth a few more years of youthful skin. So take the time!

Surgical and Non-Surgical Skin Care Treatments

There are many surgical and non-surgical treatments that are offered by spa professionals, dermatologists, and plastic surgeons for skin rejuvenation.

Here are a few non-surgical treatments you might want to consider for a more youthful glow:

✳ *Facials.* There are all types of skin rejuvenating facials. Not only are they relaxing, but they can really do great things for your skin. Try to have a professional facial every four to eight weeks.

✳ *Glycolic peels.* These can be performed on your neck, face, and chest. If you consider skin like layered bricks, the peel undoes the mortar and loosens up the goop that is clogging pores and refines fine lines. Straight glycolic peels (or un-buffered) penetrate twenty-one layers of skin, renewing the glow of a fresh face. Biolactic peels are for hyper pigmentation and those with sensitive skin. With glycolic peels, you will see immediate results.

✳ *Microdermabrasion.* This polishes and buffs skin, but does not penetrate like glycolic. A machine blasts tiny salt crystals on your skin to exfoliate the dead cells, and then vacuums them off. This can be used on your face, neck, chest, and hands. You might be a little red for an hour afterwards, but you can still exercise, swim, or even wear makeup.

the difference. Professionally applied bleach whiteners use peroxide in concentrations ranging from fifteen to thirty-five percent, while at-home products have less than twelve percent. Professionals isolate your gums, either with a protective gel or a rubber dam, before applying the peroxide. Then they use heat, a special light or a laser is directed at your teeth, to hasten the process. You might leave the office with teeth up to ten shades brighter in about an hour's time. If you have sensitive teeth, make sure the expert whitening your teeth knows. Don't eat or drink anything that would stain a white shirt for twenty-four hours after the procedure; your teeth are porous and will stain easily.

Maintaining Your Smile

Whitening starts to fade in one month, so upkeep is half the battle. If you take care of your teeth, you might be able to keep those pearly whites white for up to a year without any touchups.

* Choose toothpaste with a whitening ingredient for use once or twice a week.

* Update your daily routine. Most people don't brush for long enough. You should be putting bristle to tooth for at least two minutes each time you brush. Power brushes are great at removing surface plaque.

* Avoid foods and beverages that stain, like coffee, red juices, wine, and tea. If you can't stay away, consider using a straw so that the liquid bypasses your front teeth (but then your lip muscles are making those little lines around your lips…what's a girl to do?). Brush immediately after consuming stain-causing culprits. But be careful about brushing right after drinking soda, diet or otherwise. Research has uncovered that soda weakens the surface of your teeth and brushing within an hour of having pop can cause layers of your teeth to deteriorate. This can cause your teeth to become yellow by exposing the dentin (the layer underneath the enamel).

* Avoid foods with acid, such as those with vinegar or citrus. The acids can make your enamel more porous and more susceptible to staining.

The Skin Your Whole Body Lives In

Your face isn't the only part of you that might see some differences in its looks with age. We've been working our muscles of our bodies with exercise, but what about the changes that happens to our bodies on the outside? Things like visible veins and cellulite are enough to make any woman run screaming. But there are way to take care of these issues.

Spider veins are tiny purple veins that you can see through the skin. Most people see a fifty to ninety percent improvement in spider veins with sclerotherapy. During this

✳ Tall

Well, this one is a no brainier. Why is it that models model fashion? Because they are tall and clothes tend to look better on them, especially if they are also slim. One of my best friends, Georgia is a beautiful tall (5' 10") woman who used to model (I avoid lying out in a bikini next to her). She says there are still a few dos and don'ts, depending if your tall body has a long torso or a short one.

Dos:

- Heels or flats, depending on your outfit
- Classic basics are best

Don'ts:

- Outfits that show your stomach
- Vertical stripes and heels together

✳ Full Bottom

The goal is to find balance between your bottom and top while elongating your figure.

Dos:

- Lower cut waistbands
- Tailored jackets that flare over your hips and bottom
- Loose, straight, or slightly flared pants with fastenings on the side
- Dark colors on bottom, or vertical stripes
- Single-breasted jackets/suits
- Shoulder pads to help your shoulders balance your bottom
- Wrap dresses or slightly flared skirts that flow over your hips
- V-necklines and turtlenecks
- One-piece swimsuits with plunging cuts and wild prints
- Two-piece swimsuits with athletic style bottoms in dark colors

Don'ts:

- High waistbands
- Pleats
- Tapered to ankle pants
- Short waisted tops or jackets
- Big prints, details, or pockets on jeans
- Clinging dresses or tight pants
- Thong bikini

✳ Tummy

This is everyone's most favorite body part to work, least favorite to show. You want to draw attention to your legs or upper body with verticals or clothes that elongate your figure.

Dos:

- Hide your tummy with longer tops
- Tops/shirts that come up on the sides, scoop in the front
- Tops that focus more on the bust, less on the tummy
- Dresses that cling slightly at your hips not your waist
- Flat front pants with side fastening
- Low waist jeans, but not too low
- Jackets tailored in at the waist
- Suits with vertical lines and jackets past the waist
- One-piece swimsuits

Don'ts:

- Tanks or cropped tops
- Belts
- Gathered waist paints, shirts, dresses
- Pants with waistbands that make your tummy hang over
- Shirts tucked in
- Two-piece swimsuits

✳ Full Bust

Some like this body part to be over-emphasized. After all, it's a man magnet. However, full busts can make women look top heavy. You want to lift your breasts back into place and elongate your torso and neck.

Dos:

- Dark colored tops with wide and low necklines
- Open necklines with small lapel
- Three-quarter or longer length sleeves with flare
- Verticals above the waist
- Wraps in dresses and tops
- One- or two-piece swimsuits with V-neckline, solid color, and built-in support
- Compression sport bras

Don'ts:

- Tops with high necklines or tanks
- Boxy or loose, baggy tops
- Double breasted jackets/suits
- Wide belts
- Horizontals on top
- Go braless

Small Bust

Thank you fashion world for the wonder bra. But, don't feel bad if you're small-chested—there's a reason why you don't see models with big chests. This is because some of the best-fitted clothes are on those with less on top.

Dos:

- Tanks and capped-sleeves and halter tops
- Emphasize toned arms with sleeve-less shirts/tops
- Push-up bras
- Horizontal lines from the waist up
- Fitted jackets/suits
- Backless or low cut dresses
- Bright colors on top
- Swimsuits with skimpier bottoms or one-piece suits with all-over prints

Don'ts:

- Tube tops
- Spaghetti strap tops or dresses
- Oversized or baggy tops or dresses
- Swimsuits with full-cut bottoms and small tops

Large Thighs/Saddlebags

This is a common area where many women gain weight, usually called "saddlebags" or "thunder thighs." You can be small on top but yet have these bulges on the outer thighs giving you a pear-shaped figure. Your goal is to draw attention upward to your torso and face…so smile a lot!

Dos:

- Tops that end just above your hips
- Dark solid colors on the bottom
- A-line dresses or skirts
- Suits/jackets with big lapels, shoulder pads, three quarter in length with slight flare
- One-piece swimsuits with print on top, solid on bottom
- Wide and horizontal necklines and detailed collars that balance hips
- Pants with small waistband just above hips and flare bottoms

Don'ts:

- Tops that are boxy, baggy, or white
- Long wraps
- Small tops with big bottoms
- Two-piece swimsuits
- Pants that cut in at the ankle
- Pants with slanted pockets or pleats
- Boxy or drawstring pants or those that cinch at the waist

✱ Broad Shoulders/Small Hips

Your goal is to take attention away from your shoulders. This is the reverse problem to the pear figure.

Dos:

- V necklines, small lapels, and collars

- Single breasted jackets/suits cropped at the hips

- Dark colored tops with long sleeves

- Jackets with vertical lines and a slight flare at the waist

- Lower rise pants with pockets and detail at the waist

- One- or two-piece swimsuits

- If you wear board shorts it will balance out a smaller top

Don'ts:

- Anything that draws attention to your shoulders

- Shoulder pads

- Horizontal tops with wide cut necklines

- Double breasted jackets/suits

- Puffy sleeves or off-the-shoulder tops

- High waisted pants with wide waistbands

There isn't any body type that can't look good in the right style. Experiment with color, fabric, and texture. Don't get in a rut of wearing the same colors. Mix it up! But when in doubt, black is always safe and slimming.

Quality clothes made of better fabrics might cost a little more, but they'll wear a lot longer than cheaply made clothes. Quality is better in the long run than quantity, so go for the classic basics that will last.

When it comes to workout clothes, you want fabrics that absorb sweat and allow your body to breath. I can always tell the students in my class who feel good about their bodies…they're in the front row in colors and styles that show off all their hard working bodies. It's the students in the back row who are hiding in their big, baggy T-shirts and boxy, wide gray or black sweatpants. You can still look good while getting in shape, which will encourage you to keep coming back, as you see your body becoming stronger and more fit. Then you'll start moving up toward the front of the class.

It's up to you to defy gravity in all areas, but clothes are the easiest to start with. It's the body and skin that require more work. Find the right style for you and dress for success in every area of your life!

Learning to Accept and Appreciate Our Bodies

When you look in the mirror, do you like what you see? Do you see a person who reflects health or do you see someone who is less than healthy? We can have a distorted perception of what we see. For instance, individuals with eating disorders only see themselves as overweight—they perceive parts of their bodies unlike they really are. Sometimes there are other factors that affect our ability to accept and appreciate ourselves. Things like abuse from others or from critical loved ones. After all, if someone else is telling you how fat or ugly you are, sooner or later you start to believe it. We're hard enough on ourselves; we don't need others' negative feedback.

> *Acceptance is not submission; it is acknowledgment of the facts of a situation. Then deciding what you're going to do about it.*
>
> —Kathleen Casey Theisen

Those of us who exercise on a regular basis and eat healthy (most of the time) know when we gain even the tiniest amount of weight. Although others might not see it and think we're crazy for mentioning it, we feel it. On the other hand, there are times in our lives when life-changing events might affect our weight, body, or health. I personally have gone through many events that have had a major effect on my body and emotions. The first was the devastation of a miscarriage, which then lead to pumping my body full of fertility drugs. If you've ever experienced this, you will know that it does a big 360 on your body—not to mention all the hormones flying around like killer bees! After several attempts and failures, my emotions and body needed a break.

It takes a while to rebuild your spirits, faith, and to regain the body you once knew. One of my good friends was and is my gynecologist, Dr. Dianne Rosenberg, M.D. She watched my body change from fit to fat and tried to educate me on the effect the medication I was taking was having on my body. This is not medication that just leaves your body once you stop taking it; only over a period of time does it slowly disappear.

Needless to say, I was heavier (fifteen pounds over my usual weight), depressed, and needed to pick myself back up. The only way I knew how to do that was through exercise and surrounding myself with loving friends and family.

After two months off the medication and still heavier than what I wanted to be, my former husband told me that I was fat and because of who I am should not look the way

I did. In his mind, two months after over a year on fertility drugs, I should be back to my old self by then.

That leads me to my second big life-changing event…a divorce. Now my body was on the fast track to losing more than I ever wanted. The divorce diet is not a healthy one and in the end you'll pay for it if you allow your body to starve. With this knowledge, I did everything I could to keep feeding it good nutrition, but within a year and a half my body became a yo-yo. I lost twenty pounds (both fat and muscle) and gained twenty pounds.

I hear more women in their forties and fifties say that they have come to accept and respect themselves and others more at this age than ever before. It's not about pleasing others; it's about accepting and appreciating ourselves. Only then can you accept and appreciate others.

There is a purpose and plan for us all and, although we might not understand it the moment it happens, in time it will be revealed to us. However, it is up to us to take action and make changes. If you find yourself in an abusive relationship or around people that don't nourish your spirit and soul, then there is no way you can ever accept and appreciate yourself. If you get help or remove yourself form the unhealthy situation, you will see the difference in your attitude, health, and body. For myself, I'm so happy to be free from everyday judgment and dishonesty, and it shows through my attitude and body!

If you lead a healthy lifestyle, most likely you feel good about yourself. You like what you see, you have energy, and you're proud and accepting of your body. Those who don't exercise, eat poorly, live in a bad environment, and don't take care of their personal hygiene won't like what they see. And believe me, that shows in how they dress and conduct themselves.

Self-image sets the boundaries of individual accomplishment.
—Maxwell Maltz

One of my favorite poems is by Marlena Gutierrez, which I first read in Debra Waterhouse's book *Outsmarting the Midlife Fat Cell.* We can be so hard on ourselves…telling ourselves how much we hate our thighs or wish our butts were more like J.Lo's. Instead of always being down on our bodies, we should stop and thank them for all the wonderful things they do for us. So here is a poem—an apology to your body that I recommend you keep.

AN APOLOGY TO MY BODY

*For all the times I hated you, I hated you, said you were
"too fat," "too ugly," too anything.*

*For all the times I cried in frustration because you
didn't look like I wanted you to.*

*For all the times I put you down in my own mind
and in front of others.*

*For all the times I allowed someone to criticize you
and judge you as "not good enough."*

For all the times I thought you were awkward, graceless, clumsy.

*For all the times I tried to change you by dieting,
depriving you of true nourishment.*

For all those times, forgive me.

*Forgive me for not seeing you as the wondrous and
beautiful body you really are and always have been.*

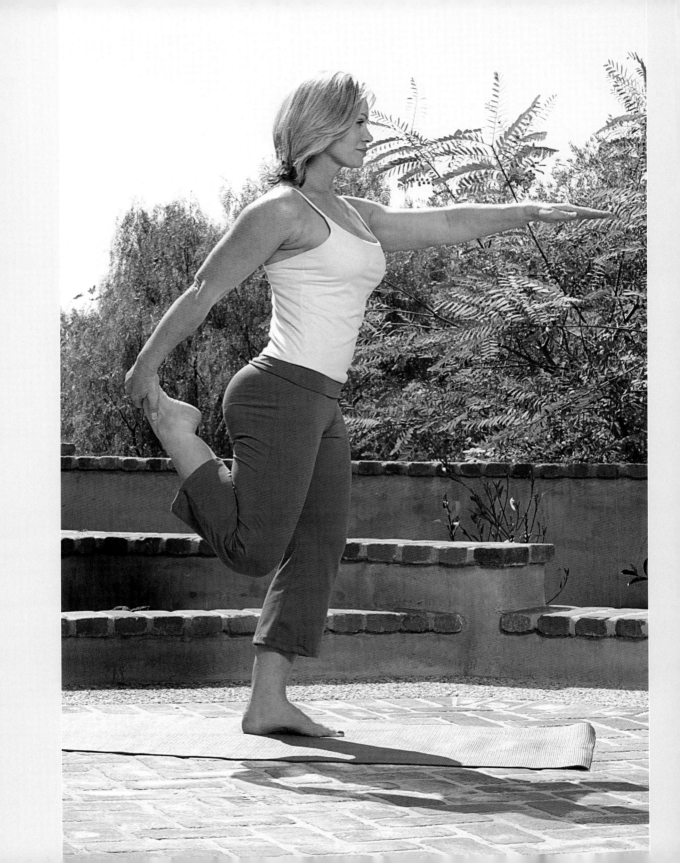

CHAPTER NINE

Women of Steel

From Bubble Butt to Buns of Steel

How did I get where I am today? From a young girl growing up on a small farm in Northern California with her two brothers and parents to a middle-aged woman living in Southern California making a living off of what her brothers would tease her for... her bubble butt!

When one door of happiness closes, another opens;
but often we look so long at the closed door that we
do not see the one which has been opened for us.

—Helen Keller

I can remember running to my bedroom and crying because my brothers and cousins would call me "bubble butt." "Your butt is so round it looks like a basketball!" they would tease. As I grew older, I would make fun of my bubble butt before anyone else could... just to let everyone know I'm very aware of my round butt. But, thanks to Beyoncé and J.Lo, I'm finally in vogue!

People e-mail me every day, mostly with questions in regards to exercise, but every once in a while I receive an e-mail that is so off the wall that I wonder if it was really meant for me. One particular e-mail read, "You should be ashamed for having butt implants. I hope that your laughable fake butt explodes and teaches you a lesson for putting poison in your body!" If I was going to have butt implants, why would I ever get them this large? Kids can say hurtful things, but when adults say them, it's just ignorance!

It wasn't until I was in college that I decided I wanted a career in fitness, but at that time the only thing that was offered was Physical Education. Aerobics was just coming of age, thanks to pioneers like Jackie Sorenson and Judi Sheppard Missett (Jazzercise).

One summer I visited family in San Diego (where I now live) and took my first aerobics class with a teacher named Mindy, who twenty years later continues to teach fitness classes and is one of my best friends. When I returned to college, I began teaching an aerobics class to other students. It was such a big hit that I had over sixty students. I taught two classes in a row to accommodate all the women who wanted to take my one-hour, high impact class. Wow! Remember the energy you had at nineteen? I added two more classes: Super Abs, which all the guys wanted as well as the gals (you gotta love that), and Hips on Down, which is what the girls wanted to work. That was the start of my career teaching fitness classes.

After graduating from California State University of Chico with a Education and a M.A. in Exercise Science, I headed south to San Diego wh career…in retail! No, that's not where I wanted to be, but every experie something you'll need to know for the future (although you might not the time).

So why was I working retail when I wanted to be teaching in a school everything I didn't learn in college…like all the different sport shoes, what they were made of, what shoe is best for which sport, and why mesh is better for sweating than leather. On the side, I would teach fitness classes at local fitness clubs, sometimes two to three a day. Of course if I tried that today, I would end up in bed for a week. In the end, I learned so much about dealing with consumers, listening to what they needed, and what products were best for which sport.

It wasn't long before I thought it might be a good idea to look into physical therapy, since there were no teaching jobs at the junior colleges. So I volunteered my time at a rehab center and learned other ways to condition a muscle…with rubber. Physical therapists where using surgical tubing and rubber bands to rehabilitate injuries. Rubber has a positive and negative resistance, meaning it has resistance (positive) when you pull as well as and on the return (negative). How much you push or pull depends on the size of the rubber tube or band and the range of motion. This experience gave me the idea to use rubber bands in my exercise classes: If they help to strengthen people with injuries, why can't they do the same for un-injured people?

This led me to my first book, *The Original Rubber Band Workout.* While working at the famous health spa (at that time they called it a "Fat Farm") the Golden Door Spa and Resort near San Diego, I meet a guest who was interested in helping me get my book published. More on that later.

The Golden Door was a beautiful resort set in Japanese style that hosted thirty-six guests for one week at a time. Once again I found myself in a job that taught me so much. Up until then, most of the people taking my exercise classes were young girls who could do hard core aerobic, high impact classes. At the Golden Door, the clients were wealthy, middle-aged, out-of-shape women who wanted to get fit in seven days and they were paying a lot of money to do it. Aerobic classes at the Golden Door are called "DeVinci classes." They are 45 minutes of aerobic dance with anywhere from eight to twelve women. Depending on their fitness level, they would be assigned to DeVinci One, Two, or Three…One being the advanced, Two intermediate, and Three beginner. I was given DeVinci Three my first week. I went from jumping, hopping, and dancing to "Whip it, Whip it Good" to "Do the Hokey Pokey."

As a fitness staff employee, it was our job to be assigned three to four women each week (men's week were limited to two weeks a year) to coordinate their fitness tests, oversee their progress, make them a take-home exercise video, and see that their week was going well. My first week on the job I got lucky…Christy Brinkley was a guest and she was assigned to me! I was so excited. She was young, beautiful, and in great shape…plus she had just fallen in love with Billy Joel and she had that "I'm in love" look (and he sent her a dozen roses every day!). When it came time to make her personal exercise video I asked what was her favorite music, so I could include it on her tape—her response? Billy Joel, of course!

Three years at the Golden Door taught me many new things about fitness, people, travel, and life. With every new experience you meet new people who might be contacts for the next chapter in your life or they might teach you more about something you thought you knew so much about. During those years, I got to travel to Japan, China, Korea, Hong Kong, Panama, and the Cayman Islands on one of the ships that the Golden Door staffs. This was where "Sit and Be Fit" was the hot class (and I thought the Hokey Pokey was slow). It was on my second trip to the Great Wall of China that I decided to stay on the ship and write my Rubber Band book. Upon returning to the Golden Door, it was that week that I meet a woman by the name of Ruth who helped find a publisher that was willing to take a chance on a no-name fitness person with a creative workout. *The Original Rubber Band Workout* was published in 1986 and is now in five different languages and continues to sell today.

Because my rubber band workout was so different, I was asked to present it at one of our industry's first fitness conference put on by International Dance Exercise Association (I.D.E.A.) in San Diego. It was a hit, and after the class I had foreigners asking me to come to their countries to teach my workout.

This is where I began working for myself and traveling all over the world, teaching other instructors my workout programs. As I continued to conduct workshops, seminars, and presentations at fitness conferences, I was approached by Steve Block, the owner of a company that made workout rubber products called Spri Products. A business marriage was created. I needed a durable rubber band that wouldn't break as easily as the bands I was using from an office supply store; he needed a fitness professional to represent his product. That was over twenty years ago, and I'm proud to say we are still working together and are great friends.

It was Steve Block who recommended me to the producer who was looking for an instructor for the workout video *Buns of Steel*. When I asked him why he suggested me, his answer was, "There is no other instructor that has Buns of Steel like yours." It was the first time I had ever heard someone refer to my buns as "Steel"…it had always been "Bubble." Twenty-two *Steel* video titles later and over ten million tapes sold, I became the Woman of Steel. Now who's laughing little brothers?

Back to reality…this "Woman of Steel" continues to have it. On the inside I do what it takes to be healthy. It's the outside that is changing, and I'm doing my best to defy gravity. But it's learning to accept the things that you cannot change and learning to love and appreciate yourself that is the important rule. For it's your soul and spirit that really project to others and go way beyond the physical person we are on the outside. It's just that most of us don't get it until we reach our forties or fifties, while others never get it. Then there are those who try to hold on to what once was. You should instead enjoy the now and what is to come.

Empowering Women

There are so many women from our past and present who are known as empowering women for the many changes they have made or are making in our society for women. Many of these women have made it easier for us women today to vote, work, make personal choices for our body, and play sports. I can't imagine not being able to make choices on what I think is right for me. Thank you ladies for your determination, commitment, and perseverance. It's because of you that I am free to be me.

The women I have listed below are, in my opinion, empowering women. They are defying the aging process through exercise, nutrition, and lifestyle choices. They have come to terms with their bodies and have learned through trial and error that life changes, as do the seasons. It is our choice to roll with the changes as the years pass by. Nothing stays the same…not even something as strong as a rock. But we can try to keep up with our bodies and what they endure with every passing decade. We can defy gravity (to a certain degree) with what we are given instead of giving up and letting those changes defy us. It is with age and the knowledge these years bring that we learn to accept the things we cannot change and change the things we can.

The women on my list have three things in common: First, they are all celebrities and find themselves constantly in the public eye. Second, they (in my opinion) have defied the aging process as women, not celebrities. The third reason…well, that's for you to figure out for yourself (don't worry, the answer is at the end of the list).

You might want to add a few names of your own favorite celebs and powerful women to this list. These are the ones that stand out in my mind. The one thing to remember is that these women don't defy gravity because of their status in society or their money. After all, it takes no money to exercise and only a little money to eat healthily and take care of your personal grooming. As I said above, it's a choice that only you can make for yourself.

Loni Anderson (actress)
Gloria Allred (attorney)
Lauren Bacall (actress)
Christie Brinkley (model)
Carol Burnett (actress)
Laura Bush (first lady)
Jackie Collins (author)
Glenn Close (actress)
Hillary Clinton (senator)
Jamie Lee Curtis (actress)
Geena Davis (actress)
Bo Derek (actress)
Chris Evertt (athlete)
Linda Evans (actress)

Peggy Flemming (athlete)
Jane Fonda (actress)
Goldie Hawn (actress)
Lauren Hutton
   (actress/model)
Iman (model)
Kate Jackson (actress)
Diane Keaton (actress)
Patty LaBelle (singer)
Christine Lahti (actress)
Cheryl Ladd (actress)
Susan Lucci (actress)
Sophia Loren (actress)
Rita Moreno (actress)

Mary Tyler Moore (actress)
Dolly Parton
   (singer/actress)
Chita Rivera
   (Broadway actress)
Dianna Ross (singer)
Diane Sawyer
   (news personality)
Susan Sarandon (actress)
Jaclyn Smith (actress)
Kathy Smith
   (fitness expert)
Meryl Streep (actress)
Barbara Streisand
   (singer/actress)

Donna Summer (singer)

Tina Turner (singer)

Raquel Welsh (actress)

Oprah Winfrey
(actress/TV show
host/media mogul)

Candace Bergen (actress)

Barbara Babcock (actress)

Anne Bancroft (actress)

Jacqueline Bisset (actress)

Faye Dunaway (actress)

Mia Farrow (actress)

Sally Field (actress)

Ali MacGraw (actress)

Shirley MacLaine (actress)

Bette Midler
(singer/actress)

Gloria Steinem
(feminist movement)

Kim Bassinger (actress)

Helen Gurley Brown
(editor of *Cosmopolitan*)

Joan Lunden (journalist)

Carly Simon (singer)

Priscilla Presley (actress)

Jane Seymore (actress)

Marlo Thomas (actress)

Sela Ward (actress)

Sigourney Weaver (actress)

After reading the list, what do you think is the third thing in common that these women have? They're all fifty years or older! Does it really take fifty years to figure out what we're made of and how to be comfortable in our own skin and body? Whether we come to accept and appreciate our bodies or not, there are a few things that most women at fifty agree on...

* Don't care so much of what others think of you. Focus on what you think of yourself.

* Take care of what's on the inside. It's more important than what's on the outside.

* Having a small group of quality friends is better then having large quantities of friends.

* Caring for our loved ones is the most important thing after taking care of ourselves.

For those of you younger than thirty-five years old reading this book, look what you have to look forward to! As you age, everything around you changes, including your own self, but remember, you have a choice. You can defy gravity or let it defy you.

Woman of Steel

Believe it or not, singing and performing is really what I thought I'd be doing in life. But after two voice surgeries and years of abuse to my vocal cords from teaching aerobics without a microphone, I had to leave this arena to others—people like my talented friend Carrie Weiland. When I first moved to San Diego, Carrie was the aerobics director where I taught. It's more than twenty years later, and she is still my boss and the director of Frogs Club One in Solana Beach, California—when she's not singing her heart out with her band.

Carrie and one of her band members, Burt Newman, wrote me a song titled "Women of Steel," which we recorded in the studios. I wanted to share this song with you because the words reflect a strong, intelligent woman that knows how to balance both mind and body!

WOMAN OF STEEL

Lyrics and music by Carrie Weiland and Burt Newman

'Xcuse me Mister may I have a word or two
   with you
As I passed by I caught your eye admiring
   the view
Don't waste my time on some worn out line
It won't work in this day and age
Sit yourself right down and I'll tell you how
Some of us women are feelin' today

You got to be strong both body and mind
You got to take control, but very lady-like
Being a Super Woman just won't do

Chorus

I got to be a woman of steel
A little tough, a lot of love and in-between
A hair-fluffin', knows-her-stuff woman
I got to be a woman of steel

You might think I need a man to make my
   life complete
That's not so true, I don't need you, to stand
   on my own two feet
I'm a CEO with a PhD and a B-O-D-Y to match
And when it comes to lovin' let me tell
   you somethin'
I'm the best that you ever had

Now I can look good in a sequin dress
And still know how to get a little respect
Being a Super Woman just won't do

Chorus

I got to be a woman of steel
A little tough, a lot of love and in-between
A man-huggin', knows-her-stuff woman
I got to be a woman of steel

Bridge

Survivin' in this world today
Takes all of your strength
We live so fast and good lovin'
Sometimes can't keep the pace
A man like you might be confused
On how to play his part
Give that woman of steel a little TLC
And she'll open up her heart

'Xcuse me darlin' may I have a word or two
   with you
You see I've been a woman long enough
To know your point of view
In this day and age you'd think a man
Could understand how we all feel
You got to know that deep down inside
Every woman is a woman of steel

Chorus

You got to be a woman of steel
A little tough, a lot of love and in-between
An ain't she somethin', knows-her-stuff woman
Got to be a woman of steel
A hair-fluffin', man-huggin', ain't-she-some-
thin', knows-her-stuff woman
Woman of steel

Resources and Recommended Reading

911 Beauty Secrets. Diane Irons. Sourcebooks, Inc., 1999.

Before The Change Taking Charge of Your Perimenopause. Ann Louise Gittleman Ph.D. HarperCollins Publishers, Inc., 1998.

Defying Age. Dr. Miriam Stoppard. London: DK, 2003. First American Edition, 2004.

Fight Fat after Forty. Pamela Peeke M.D., M.P.H. New York: Penguin Putnam Inc., 2000.

Fit Not Fat at 40 Plus. Editors of Prevention for Women. Rodale, 2002.

Fit & Well. Thomas D Fahey Ph.D., Paul M. Insel, and Walton T. Roth. California: Mayfield Publishing Company, 1999.

Get With the Program: Guide to Fast Food & Family Restaurants. Bob Greene. New York: Simon & Schuster, 2004.

Lower Your Fat Thermostat. Dennis Remington M.D., Garth Fisher Ph.D., and Edward Parent Ph.D. Utah: Vitality House International Inc., 1983.

Meditations for Women Who Do Too Much. Anne Wilson Schaef. San Francisco: Harper, 1990.

Outsmarting the Female Fat Cell. Debra Waterhouse. New York: Warner, 1992.

Secrets of Style. Lisa Arbetter and InStyle Editors. New York: Melcher Media, Inc., 2003.

Strong Women Stay Young. Miriam E. Nelson, PH.D.. New York: Bantam Books, 1997.

SuperFoods. Steven Pratt, M.D. and Kathy Matthews. New York: Harper Collins Publishers, Inc., 2004.

Super Nutrition for Menopause. Anne L. Gittleman. New York: Pocket Books, 1993.

The Book of Positive Quotations. John Cook. Minneapolis, MN: Fairview Press, 1996.

The Female Power Within. Marilyn Graman and Maureen Walsh. New York: Life Works Books, 2002.

The G.I. Glycemic Index Diet. Rick Gallop. New York: Workman Publishing, 2002.

The Original Rubber Band Workout. Tamilee Webb M.A. New York: Workman Publishing, 1986.

The Pilates Back Book. Tia Stanmore. Fair Winds Press, 2002.

The Pocket Stylist. Kendall Farr. Penguin Group, 2004.

The Ultimate Body: 10 Perfect Workouts for Women. Liz Neporent M.A. New York: The Ballantine Book, 2003.

The 60-Minute Meltdown: Fight Cellulite and Win. Thomas Fahey Ph.D. Fitness RX for Women Magazine, 2003.

Total Pilates. Ann Crowther with Helena Petre. Harper Collins Publishers, 2003.

WalkFit™ For A Better Body. Kathy Smith. New York: Time Warner Company, 1994.

Weight Training for Women. Thomas D. Fahey and G. Hutchinson. Mountain View, CA: Mayfield Publishing, 1992.

What Not to Wear. Susannah Contantine and Trinny Woodall. New York: Riverhead Books, 2002.

Women's Bodies, Women's Wisdom. Christiane Northrup M.D. New York: Bantam Books, 2002.

Workouts for Dummies. Tamilee Webb M.A. New York: IDG Books, 1998.

Yoga Beats The Blues. Donna Raskin. Fair Winds Press, 2003.

Wake Up to Life. Jean Pierre Marques. www. evolutioninhealth.com.

Useful
Contact Information

Tamilee Webb
Webb International Inc.
7031 Calle Portone
Rancho Santa Fe, CA 92091
www.tamileewebb.com

Spri Products Inc.
1600 Northwind Blvd.
Libertyville, IL 60048
800.222.7774
www.spriproducts.com

Frogs Club One
511 South Hwy 101
Solana Beach, CA 92075
www.clubone.com

IDEA Health & Fitness Association
10455 Pacific Center Court
San Diego, CA 92121-4339
800.999.4332
www.ideafit.com

Ultra Fit Nutrition
PO Box 489
Solana Beach, CA 92075
www.ultrafitnutrition.com

American Council on Exercise
4851 Paramount Drive
San Diego, CA 92123
800.825.3636
www.acefitness.com

Debra Waterhouse (author/speaker)
www.waterhousepublishion.com

Carrie Weiland (singer/songwriter)
315 South Coast Hwy 101 #64
Encinitas, CA 92024
www.carrieweiland.com

Thomas Fahey, Ed. D., Ph.D.
California State University, Chico
Chico, CA 95929

Goldhil Media
5284 Adolfo Road
Camarillo, CA 93012

www.naturaljourneys.com

Clothing Resources

www.kos-usa.com
www.marika.com

Acknowledgments

To Fair Winds Press: This book was conceived by one of your editors (Donna Raskin) while working out. Thank you, Donna, for letting your creative mind come up with "Defy Gravity" and having the confidence in me to be the fitness personality to share with you and other women at the forty-something threshold what I've found…how to keep it (or at least keep it from sagging). You have helped me get back into my groove with a title that has inspired me. Thanks to all the others at Fair Winds Press, including Holly Schmidt and Rhiannon Soucy.

To My Students at Frogs who come and exercise with me every week and share their personal experiences with their changing bodies: Thank you for telling me what it's really like at fifty, fifty-five, and sixty and being there to try out every new exercise before it goes to video or DVD…you're much better than mice!

To My Girlfriends: This one is big because without my friends who were there for me during trying times to pick me up, dust me off, and point me back in the right direction…I'm not sure where I would have ended up. It is all of you who gave me strength when I thought my world had fallen apart, who helped me swim when I wanted to drown and opened my eyes to see the real beauty of making it to the other side. These are women who make me proud to be a woman…Lee Block, Shanhaz Brown, Karen Creelman, Diane Colyer, Teresa Cundiff, Candy Drolson, Sue DeSimone, Sonia Desormeaux, Georgia Goldberg, Gita Gendloff, Sally Ray Gunther, Kris Gelbert, Dennis Hendricks, Rosemarie Houston, Michelle Iafrate, Jessica Janc, Mary Kay Jordon, Carolyn Lords, Mindy Marinos, Kelley Martinez, Darcy Micco Pace, Jeanie McCarthy, Cindy Mort, Wendy Mosley, Helen Nordan, Honey Novak, Yvonne Ouellette, Gayle Paddison, Debbie Rider, Megan Ring, Dianne Rosenberg, Penny Sarver, Karen Silvas, Carolyn Singer, Rachel Tung, Debra Wood, Carrie Weiland, and Mikki Williams.

To The Bridges Country Club: Thank you, Ani Dumas, for supporting me on this project in getting some of the most beautiful photos for the book done here at the Bridges and Ken Ayors to approve it. You make living and exercising at the Bridges a delight.

To Marika and KOS: Thank you to both companies for providing me with the beautiful workout clothes for the shoot of this book. They are perfect for the forty-plus woman.

To Neala Moch: My most important instructor for my skin care program, thank you for helping me keep my skin healthy and beautiful and for your professional input into the skincare chapter of *Defy Gravity Workout.*

To Thomas Fahey, Ed. D, Ph. D.: Thanks to you, I'm able to continue my education with your on-going articles and research in the wonderful world of health and fitness. I'm proud to have been a student of yours and all the other professors at California State University, Chico.

To Goldhil Media: Gary and Debbie Goldman and Dwight Hilton along with all the staff at Goldhil Media and Natural Journeys, as well as Andrea Ambandos, the Queen producer/director of most great fitness videos. Thank you all for believing in my workouts and producing my videos/DVDs for others to enjoy.

To Cheryl Fenton: Although we only know each other through e-mails and the phone, I feel like we have traveled the world with all the back and forth writing we have done. I couldn't have written it without you, girl. Don't be scared after writing and reading *Defy Gravity Workout.* Just take good care of yourself and changes will be kind to you.

To Allen Penn & Bevan Walker: I never had so much fun on a photo shoot. Thanks for turning two working days shooting for this book into two fun days with breakfast included. Great photos guys!

And last but of course never least…to my two dogs **Kassie & Corky** for their endless love, hugs, and kisses. You both were very patient waiting for your walks as I finished just one more chapter…you deserve more treats. To my special friend **Matt Grenfell,** who helped me ride the waves when I could not surf but knew I had it in me to complete the journey…thank you!

About the Author

Tamilee Webb, M.A., is the star of the *Buns of Steel* video series which has sold over 10 million copies. She is the author of *The Original Rubber Band Workout* (sold in six countries and translated into five languages), *Step-Up-Fitness*, and *Workout for Dummies*. Tamilee has appeared on many TV shows and in several magazines.

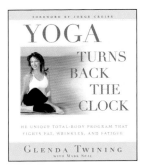

Also from Fair Winds Press

YOGA TURNS BACK THE CLOCK
by Glenda Twining with Mark Seal
ISBN: 1-59233-006-1
$19.95/£12.99/$28.95 CAN
Paperback; 192 pages
Available wherever books are sold

There Is a Magic Formula for Staying Young—Yoga!

You can be as toned, energized, and beautiful as you were in your twenties—or more so! Yoga practitioners have long known the secrets to looking and feeling young. Now you can harness the amazing power of this ancient art to fight flab and rejuvenate every part of your body with the energizing routines in this book.

Through simple step-by-step instructions and easy-to-follow full-color photos, Glenda Twining shows you the miracle of anti-aging yoga. She has helped hundreds of people turn back the clock with her unique program, and you can be next!

You'll learn:
- why 30 minutes is all it takes to transform your body
- how yoga works to rejuvenate your entire body from the inside out
- simple stretches you can do at home to fight fat and feel younger

Glenda Twining is a yoga instructor and fitness expert. Certified as a fitness specialist by the Cooper Institute for Aerobics Research, she lives and works in Dallas, Texas.